Deember 1993.

Inlays, Crowns and Bridges

Inlays, Crowns and Bridges
A Clinical Handbook

Fifth edition

Leslie C Howe BDS, FDS RCS

Wimpole Street, London
Department of Conservative Dental Surgery, United Medical and Dental Schools of Guy's and
St. Thomas's Hospitals, University of London

George F Kantorowicz BSc, BDS

Formerly Senior Lecturer in Conservative Dental Surgery, United Medical and Dental Schools
of Guy's and St. Thomas's Hospitals, University of London
Honorary Consultant Dental Surgeon, Lewisham and North Southwark Health Authority and
The Royal Dental Hospital School of Dental Surgery, University of London

Adrian C Shortall DDS, BDS, FDS RCPS, FFD RCSI

Senior Lecturer in Conservative Dentistry, The School of Dentistry, University of Birmingham
Honorary Consultant in Restorative Dentistry, South Birmingham Health Authority

David S Shovelton BSc, BDS, FDS RCS

Emeritus Professor of Conservative Dentistry, University of Birmingham
Honorary Consultant in Conservative Dentistry, South Birmingham Health Authority

Edited by
George F Kantorowicz

Wright

Wright
An imprint of Butterworth-Heinemann Ltd
Linacre House, Jordan Hill, Oxford OX2 8DP

R A MEMBER OF THE REED ELSEVIER GROUP

OXFORD LONDON GUILDFORD BOSTON
MUNICH NEW DELHI SINGAPORE SYDNEY
TOKYO TORONTO WELLINGTON

First published 1963
Second edition 1970
Third edition 1979
Reprinted 1981
Fourth edition 1985
Fifth edition 1993

British Library Cataloguing in Publication Data

Inlays, Crowns and Bridges. – 5 Rev. ed
  I. Kantorowicz, George F.
  617.675

ISBN 0 7236 2351 1

Library of Congress Cataloguing in Publication Data

Inlays, crowns and bridges/Leslie C. Howe . . . [et al.]: edited by
  George F. Kantorowicz. – 5th ed.
  p. cm.
  Includes bibliographical references and index.
  ISBN 0 7236 2351 1
  1. Inlays (Dentistry) 2. Crowns (Dentistry) 3. Bridges
  (Dentistry) I. Howe, Leslie C. II. Kantorowicz, George F.
  [DNLM: 1. Crowns. 2. Denture, Partial. 3. Inlays. WU 515 I56
  1993]
  RK666. I55 1993
  617.6'92– dc20
                                                    93–14003
                                                    CIP

Composition by R. H. Services, Welwyn, Hertfordshire
Printed and bound by Printeksa, Spain.

Contents

Preface to the first edition

This book deals with the clinical procedures for preparing and fitting inlays, crowns, and bridges. It is intended for the senior dental student and for the practitioner who wishes to embark upon more advanced operative procedures. A knowledge of routine conservative dentistry is therefore assumed.

A certain amount of dogmatism is inevitable in a short book, but the methods described are ones which have been proved in practice. Also, they are methods which have been taught to students over a period of years. Descriptions of other techniques will be found in the larger textbooks, but the authors feel that it is helpful for the student to have a concise handbook for easy reference to the techniques most usually employed.

In writing any book it is inevitable that the experience, ideas, and writings of many people are consulted. We have drawn freely from sources of information which are too numerous to acknowledge individually and we are indebted to many friends and colleagues for their help and encouragement.

We wish to thank particularly Dr R A Cawson, Mr J R Grundy, Professor Alexander B MacGregor, Professor H M Pickard, and Mr N Livingstone Ward for reading the manuscript and for their helpful criticisms and suggestions.

We also wish to thank Professor E L Hampson for permission to use an idea from his book for *Fig.* 23 A; Dr K D Jørgensen for permission to reproduce *Fig.* 1; Professor S Makinson and the Editor of the *British Dental Journal* for permission to reproduce *Fig.* 152; and Mr D M Watt for permission to reproduce *Table* III.

Our thanks for their cheerful perseverance go to Miss G Crockett, Mrs B Curtis, and Miss M Hunt, who have typed *many* drafts of the manuscript.

We wish to place on record our sincere thanks to Dr N L Bucky, our illustrator. His enthusiasm and skill in understanding dental problems and interpreting them so clearly have made the line drawings a very important feature of this book.

Last, but by no means least, we should like to thank our wives. They have tolerated our numerous conferences with remarkable equanimity.

London,
April, 1963

G F Kantorowicz

Preface to the fifth edition

The first edition of this handbook was published thirty years ago. At that time the objective of the authors was to provide a short, simple handbook, suitable for senior dental students and practitioners, dealing with the principles of making inlays, crowns and bridges. Laboratory techniques were not included.

There have been many changes in materials and techniques during the intervening years, and especially since the publication of the fourth edition. The main change, however, is that there are now two new authors, both experienced clinicians and teachers, who have introduced new ideas and attitudes. All these changes are reflected in this new edition, which has been completely revised and every chapter extensively rewritten.

The aim of the authors of this edition remains the same as that of previous editions, and for this reason the book continues to contain a certain amount of dogmatism in describing methods that have been taught to students successfully. It is not suggested that the methods described are the only ones suitable for each procedure, and descriptions of other techniques can be found in larger textbooks, but the authors believe that it is helpful to have a concise handbook describing techniques that are tried and trusted.

Once again we have drawn freely from the experience and ideas of many of our colleagues, too numerous to be acknowledged individually, but we are indebted to them all for their help.

New line drawings have been provided by Miss Sarah Davenport while Dr A Atta, Dr R Palmer, Mr M Mars, Mr R Marx, Dr F J Fisher, Mr A S Britton, Mr D H Roberts, Mr A McCullock, Mr C Allen and Ultradent Products Ltd. are amongst colleagues who have allowed us to use some of their material and photographs. We are grateful to them.

Finally, we wish to express our gratitude to those dental technicians with whom we have worked over the years, who have provided the highly skilled laboratory cooperation needed in inlay crown and bridge work.

London,   G F Kantorowicz
December, 1992

Chapter 1

General principles

Introduction

Why are inlays, crowns and bridges made? In the case of gold inlays one reason is because gold is stronger than other restorative materials and can be used in thin sections without danger of fracture. This toughness, combined with its accuracy of fabrication and its lack of corrosion, makes it a unique restorative material. The appearance of gold is preferable to that of amalgam. Ceramic and composite inlays give a still better appearance and, in addition, strengthen weakened cusps by bonding to tooth tissue.

Crowns are usually indicated for grossly damaged teeth or when the appearance of a tooth is to be improved (Figure 1.1). The main advantage of bridges is that they avoid the need for wearing partial dentures which, however well made, must be removed regularly for cleaning. A bridge, on the other hand, restores appearance and function and becomes part of the patient's dentition (Figure 1.2).

We are in an era of exciting changes in materials and techniques, but these newer procedures must stand the test of time before they can be incorporated into standard teaching. Hopefully this will occur and some newer and less well established techniques and materials are included in this book where appropriate and when, in the opinion of the authors, it seems

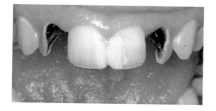

a

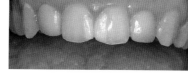

b

Figure 1.1 (a) Badly broken-down upper lateral incisors. (b) Post crowns placed after endodontic treatment, restoring function and appearance

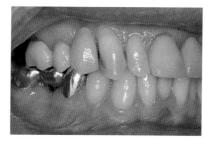

Figure 1.2 Metal ceramic bridge replacing upper right first premolar and all-gold bridge replacing lower right first molar

probable that they will prove their worth.

There is continued growth in the use of implants to support both single-tooth replacements and bridges. Whilst the techniques for implant retained restorations are outside the remit for this book, it is worth remembering that they are a possible treatment option.

Implant procedures have been proposed for many years but it is only with the development of the Branemark system (Nobelpharma, UK) in Sweden that they have become generally acceptable and scientifically researched. The important factors in successful implants are that the implant fixture becomes fully 'osseo-integrated' into the remaining jaw bone. This is achieved by a careful surgical technique to ensure an exact fit for a sterile, biocompatible titanium fixture. This is allowed to remain unloaded and fully covered by mucosa for at least 6 months, during which time the surrounding bone grows around the fixture and stabilizes the implant.

A second surgical phase uncovers the head of the fixture, and the restoration is produced and then screwed to the embedded fixture. Restorations can be single crowns, bridges or even replace full dentures with full arch bridges if enough fixtures have been placed.

The advantages of the technique are obvious: the ability to replace teeth without involvement of adjacent teeth and their preparation. This is particularly advantageous in the distal extension situation or where abutment teeth are post crowns because the presence or quality of suitable abutment teeth is not a consideration.

The limitations of implant techniques are firstly, the need for adequate bone to be present both in quantity, to allow for long fixtures, and quality; compact bone being preferred to cancellous bone. This obviously limits the use of implants, for example, in the upper molar region due to the maxillary sinus. Secondly, surgery is involved and this discourages many patients. Thirdly, the techniques are very costly and time-consuming, and finally, as with any technique, there is no guarantee of 100% success. The patient and dentist must carefully weigh up the advantages and disadvantages.

In general, advanced restorative procedures are indicated only when the patient is well-motivated and cooperative, and when the mouth is healthy with well-controlled caries and periodontal disease.

Before any treatment is undertaken it is necessary to establish a diagnosis of the dental state and to decide what, if any, treatment should be provided. A diagnosis can only be established after taking a careful history. It is important to allow patients adequate time to talk about their wishes so far as the mouth is concerned and explore their objectives in seeking advanced dental treatment. What are their wishes in relation to improvement in appearance or function, and what expectations do they have of what can be achieved? This should be followed by undertaking a full dental examination, including the provision of any necessary radiographs and study casts.

Consideration of general factors

1. *Age*
Although age provides no absolute barriers to the provision of crowns, they are generally avoided for the very young patient because of the possible

danger to the pulp of extensive conservative procedures and of the likelihood of subsequent trauma to the mouth during childhood activities. Furthermore, eruption will gradually expose the gingival margin of the preparation, which may spoil the appearance of an anterior crown.

Occasionally, however, crowns for young patients are necessary, for example when severe hypoplasia or gross loss of tooth substance makes a child sensitive about poor dental appearance.

Caution should be exercised with elderly patients where gingival recession may make it difficult, if not impossible, to place the margin of the crown close to the gingivae. A satisfactory appearance may sometimes be obtained by placing the crown margin at the cementum–enamel junction. Periodontal disease in this age group may shorten the anticipated life of a crowned tooth and thereby influence the choice of material for the crown if the prognosis is poor.

In certain circumstances, for example in patients with hypodontia, cleft palate or haemophilia, every effort should be made to avoid extractions even when circumstances are otherwise unfavourable.

2. *Periodontal condition*
The condition of the supporting structures of the tooth must be satisfactory before crown or bridge work is undertaken. Furthermore, advanced conservative procedures are indicated only for patients whose oral hygiene is good.

3. *The completeness of the dentition*
The loss of a number of teeth is generally an indication of past neglect or high caries susceptibility. For such patients, the provision of a denture or addition to an existing one is usually preferable to advanced conservation. Exceptions may be made for suitable patients. For example, six anterior teeth may be present in an otherwise edentulous jaw, but their appearance may be marred by one of them. A crown for this tooth would allow the patient to keep the six teeth and be fitted with a partial denture replacing the posterior teeth. Another example is that of a posterior tooth crowned to provide a suitable abutment for a partial denture. In some instances it may be advantageous to unite a number of teeth by crowns in order to provide the most satisfactory support for the denture.

The concept of the 'shortened dental arch' should not be forgotten. This suggests that if complete arches can be achieved from second premolar to second premolar, both upper and lower, it may be in the patient's best interests to concentrate all resources on these teeth rather than attempt to conserve badly involved molars and, at the same time, provide a lower standard of treatment for the rest of the dentition.

4. *Caries experience*
Both past and present caries experiences are relevant to the planning of restorative treatment. The need for a patient to bring caries incidence under control is paramount, whilst failure to control sugar consumption may lead to restorations failing within a comparatively short time, even with reasonably good oral hygiene.

Saliva flow should be considered, because a significant reduction reduces natural cleansing and increases the liability to caries.

5. *Tooth wear*

Throughout life some degree of tooth wear may be expected but in some patients excessive wear may occur, often at a relatively early age. It is important to diagnose the onset of this condition relatively early. The cause can then be investigated and, if found, steps taken to prevent further deterioration. The condition should be reviewed and, when necessary, restorations provided to maintain the vertical dimension or, in cases of extreme wear, to increase it.

6. *Attitude of the patient*

The majority of patients to whom the purpose of crown work is explained become keenly interested in this form of treatment. Those who lack interest and refuse to accept the role they must play in the control of dental disease or who are unwilling to cooperate during the preparation of crowns are generally not suitable for advanced conservation. Highly nervous individuals may also be unsuitable on temperamental grounds, because they make this exacting work difficult or impossible. Furthermore, the planning of advanced restorative procedures must consider the prognosis for the whole dentition.

A failure of the patient to control dental plaque must be considered a contra-indication to ambitious restorative plans. This does not mean that the patient is abandoned but that a less ambitious plan, which allows several fallback positions to be adopted, is chosen.

Clinical assessment of the individual tooth

1. *Vitality*

Teeth damaged by caries or trauma must be tested for vitality. Ideally, an electric pulp tester should be used and comparisons made with the reactions of adjacent and contra-lateral teeth. If root canal treatment is necessary, the tooth is usually only suitable for a post crown. The natural crown will be weakened by loss of dentine when access is made to the root canal, and further weakened if a jacket crown preparation is cut.

2. *Mobility*

The mobility of any tooth to be restored must be tested and compared with that of adjacent teeth. The underlying cause of tooth mobility should be identified and treated so that the prognosis of the tooth can be determined before the decision is made to proceed with a restoration.

3. *Local gingival condition*

If the gingival tissues have been affected by plaque from carious cavities or the rough edges of restorations, they must be treated and allowed to heal before final tooth preparation is attempted. This is important because the treatment usually results in some gingival recession, which may reveal the margins of the restoration and spoil its appearance.

4. *Occlusion*

The occlusion must be checked in intercuspal, lateral and protrusive excursions, particularly looking for prematurities, to assess the clearance to be gained during tooth preparation. If less than 1 mm of clearance can be achieved, an onlay or a crown with a metal occlusal surface should be considered. In addition, some judgement should be made of the occlusal force likely to be borne by the restoration during function. Clearly defined wear facets are often an indication of heavy parafunctional loads that will be exerted on a restoration.

5. *Relationship to adjacent teeth*

It is tempting to rush into correcting the appearance caused by a malpositioned tooth. A malpositioned tooth may be overlapping, spaced, proclined, retroclined or rotated. Some caution is indicated to ensure that not only can sufficient tooth be removed to correct the appearance but, in addition, sufficient tooth tissue to accommodate the crown material. If both these objectives can be achieved without endangering the pulp, and leaving enough tooth to provide a resistant and retentive preparation, then it is safe to proceed. The space available within the dental arch for an overlapped tooth may be so small that any restoration would look odd. It is wise to be aware of this before the preparation and to advise the patient of the final appearance.

6. *Radiographic investigation*

A radiograph should always be taken before the preparation is started (Figure 1.3). The information required from this is:

a. The size and position of the pulp.
b. The gingival and pulpal extent of any caries or restoration present in the tooth.
c. The condition of the supporting structures of the tooth as judged by the appearance of the alveolar crest and continuity of the lamina dura, especially in the apical region.

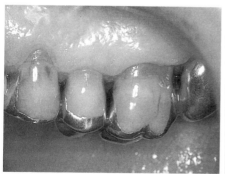
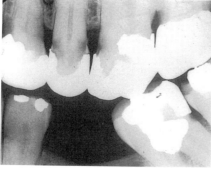

a *b*

Figure 1.3 (a) Clinical examination alone will not always reveal all caries. (b) The bite-wing radiograph reveals secondary caries beneath restorations

7. *Study casts*

Alginate impressions of the upper and lower jaws are taken at the time of examination of the patient. Study casts from these may serve the following purposes:

a. Further assessment of the occlusion.
b. Anticipated difficulties with preparations may be 'rehearsed' on the study cast.
c. Temporary crowns may be made on these casts in the laboratory. Study casts used for these procedures are certainly invaluable if multiple crowns are planned.
d. It is sometimes helpful to prepare a diagnostic wax-up on a study cast for the patient to assess the final appearance before embarking on tooth preparation.

8. *Appearance*

Possible problems with the final appearance of a crown can be foreseen in some instances at the clinical examination. For example, the restoration of a single central incisor presents a daunting challenge to the most experienced operator with first-class technical support. This difficulty is compounded if the teeth are very light in shade, opaque, or both. Thin teeth with translucent incisal edges are also very difficult to match.

9. *Photographs*

Some record of both the pre-operative and post-operative condition of the teeth and adjacent tissues is important. Photographs can form a valuable part of this record and the use of a simple and reliable photographic technique should be considered.

The diagnosis is followed by a treatment plan or plans, which should be discussed with the patient before any operative work is undertaken. Treatment plans should have the objective of achieving a healthy mouth for some years, thereby contributing to prevention as well as restoration of the mouth.

The patient must be given an estimate of the time involved; not only the total time but also the intervals between appointments and the probable length of appointments, which may be prolonged if complex work is to be undertaken. In many instances an estimate of the cost will also be required at this stage.

Throughout this book mention is made of the importance of good plaque control and well-maintained oral hygiene. It must be stressed that procedures such as inlays, crowns and bridges are likely to fail if the periodontal tissues are unhealthy and oral hygiene is not maintained at a high level. The operator must, therefore, make sure that the patient understands the importance of oral hygiene and is capable and willing to maintain it.

Necessary pre-operative periodontal treatment must be completed before the restorative procedures are begun. Healthy periodontal tissues are a prerequisite of good inlay, crown and bridge work. Periodic checks are necessary and encouragement, with further instructions for the patient, are also helpful.

Operative procedures

In this book, preparations using rotational instruments at low and high speeds are described. The term 'low speed' will refer to those instruments that operate at less than 25 000 rpm; 'high speed' will refer to speeds between 25 000 rpm and 100 000 rpm; and for speeds above 100 000 rpm, the term 'ultra-speed' will be used.

Most of the vibration frequencies of the ultra-speed instruments, such as the air turbine, are above the threshold of perception and do not therefore cause discomfort. But cutting dentine is painful, however efficiently it is done, and an air–water spray may cause pain in the lower quadrant while treating an anaesthetized upper quadrant.

The need for adequate cooling, however, cannot be overemphasized because without it the pulp can be quickly and severely damaged. Therefore an air–water spray must be used for all cavity preparations where the instrument speed is above 3000 rpm.

Ultra-speed instruments have made easier the tedious removal of sound tooth substance in the preparation of cavities and crowns. The use of ultra-speed instruments is, therefore, advocated for the majority of the work in tooth preparation. There are two aspects to finishing the preparation of teeth. One is the refinement of intracoronal detail and the other is finishing the cavo-surface angles. Sharp burs running at low speed are recommended for the first of these, and 30-bladed finishing burs or ultra-fine diamond instruments used at ultra-speed or 40 000 rpm are suggested for the second. This technique has been shown to produce excellent margins with little danger of overcutting. In all instances finishing should be done with great care because peripheral fit of the restoration depends largely on this phase of tooth preparation. Also, many otherwise good preparations are spoilt by inadvertent overcutting during finishing procedures.

This book generally describes only one method for each operative procedure, but this does not imply that the technique described is the only one possible. The method chosen in each instance, however, is one that has been found over the years to be successful even in the hands of relatively inexperienced operators. For this reason it is suggested that those who have little experience of advanced conservative procedures might, with advantage, use the techniques described in the first instance. After gaining more experience, however, each clinician will develop an individual range of techniques that are most suitable.

It must be emphasized that all advanced operative techniques demand skill from the operator and the full cooperation of the patient. Attention to detail and the utmost patience are essential. There are few, if any, short cuts that will not detract from the quality and durability of completed restorations. Equipment and instruments must be of adequate standard. Lighting of the operative field is of the greatest importance if fatigue and errors are to be avoided. Magnification ($2\times$ or $3\times$) is a useful aid in ensuring that preparations are shaped as accurately as possible, which is important if restorations are to be retentive and well-fitting.

Definitions

Cavo-surface angle   An angle formed by the junction of the wall of a cavity with the surface of a tooth.

A point angle   An angle formed at the point where three cavity walls meet.

A line angle   An angle formed at the junction of two cavity walls.

Axial wall   A wall in the long axis of a tooth.

Pulpal wall   A wall occlusal to the pulp and in a plane at right angles to the long axis of a tooth.

Protection of the pulp during operative procedures

Rotary instruments generate heat during the preparation of a tooth and precautions are necessary to prevent a rise in temperature. The heat must be dissipated before it can cause discomfort to the patient or damage to the pulp.

It has been shown in many studies that there may be a considerable rise in temperature of the pulp during cutting or grinding of dentine and enamel unless adequate coolants are used. Because of the problem when large quantities of water are used to cool teeth during conservative procedures, the use of air as a coolant has, from time to time, been advocated. It has been amply demonstrated that air alone is not as efficient for restricting the rise in pulpal temperature. It has also been shown that the dehydration of dentine caused by an air jet can, of itself, cause considerable pulpal damage. It is, therefore, stressed that when using any instrument, rotating at 3000 rpm or above, an adequate air–water spray should always be used.

A handpiece capable of producing two or more jets should be used because a single jet does not always reach the working point of the instrument. Unless an adequate spray is used, there is a serious risk of irreparable damage to the pulp, particularly if it has been previously damaged by caries, filling materials or earlier cavity preparation. An air–water spray is preferable to a water jet because its cooling ability is greater for a given volume of water. It also helps to avoid the possibility of a dry, uncooled area immediately around the rotating bur. It is important to use light and intermittent pressure during tooth preparation in order to minimize heat production.

Another factor in pulp protection is the amount of dentine removed. It appears that the more closely the preparation approaches the pulp, the greater is the degree of pulp damage, both during tooth preparation and in response to subsequent procedures, including lining and cementation. It is also likely that the more extensive the preparation the greater is the degree of trauma caused to the pulp. In the absence of infection, damage to the pulp will normally be repaired. However, scarring in the pulp as a result of repair will interfere with the nervous and vascular supply to the tissue. Long-term follow-up has indicated that pulpal necrosis and periapical lesions may develop in a small proportion (up to 10%) of teeth provided with extensive cast restorations. Care is always indicated and, for these reasons, only the minimum amount of tooth substance should be removed that is consistent with the prevention of further caries, retention of the restoration, and the strength of the material to be used.

Materials

Gold
Dental gold alloys can be cast in thin veneers that are strong enough to resist the occlusal forces and tough enough not to fracture under repeated impact. The high cost of gold has led to a search for alternative, cheaper casting alloys and the development of more sophisticated semi-precious and non-precious alloy combinations. There is much research in this area and an alternative with all the merits of the high-gold alloys but at a lower cost may be developed in the future. At present non-precious and semi-precious alloys may be used, but they have a number of disadvantages and can only really compete with the high-gold alloys on cost.

Where appearance of natural teeth is important the gold may sometimes be restricted to the non-visible parts of the clinical crown as a partial veneer crown.

Porcelain
Dental porcelains are essentially glassy materials whose main constituents are feldspar, quartz and kaolin. Porcelain is brittle but it is stable, it does not change colour in time, is not affected by the oral fluids and it can be produced in various shades. This is why it has been used for decades as the most suitable material for tooth-coloured crowns. No other material can match it when a good appearance is crucial. Porcelain crowns are usually restricted to the anterior regions but can be used in the premolar regions when the occlusion is favourable. However, in these situations it is advisable to use an occlusal thickness of material of about 1.5 mm.

Table 1.1 Casting alloys

Type	Approximate carat value	ADA specification Brinell hardness*	Proportional limit* (Newtons/mm)	Indications
I Soft	22	40–75	69	Class V inlays
II Medium	20	70–100	138	Two-surface inlays
III Hard	18	90–140	172	Onlays and inlays opposed by heavy occlusal forces. Veneer crowns and retainers opposed by average occlusal forces
IV Extra hard	18	140+	275–480	Thin veneers, thin cuspal covers, and thin pontic sections opposed by heavy occlusal forces
Gold Ceramic		130–160		Full crowns, thin veneers, bridge work
Nickel–chrome		360–370	900	
Cobalt–chromium		350	1000	

* The variation within the ranges depends on the heat treatment of the alloy.

Metal–ceramics

Porcelain can be bonded to a variety of alloys, including those with a high content of precious metals, others with a lower precious metal content and base metal alloys containing nickel and chromium.

The ability to combine the strength of metal with the appearance of porcelain superseded the use of plastic (acrylic crowns or facings) which, although useful in their time, suffered from wear and discoloration. The main reasons for using metal–ceramic crowns are similar to those for porcelain crowns but metal–ceramic crowns are more versatile, stronger and can be used as bridge retainers.

Stabilization of the mouth

It is stressed that advanced restorative procedures should normally be undertaken only when the mouth is healthy and any disease processes have been arrested or remedied. For some patients it may be necessary to undertake preliminary phases of treatment to stabilize the condition of the mouth before proceeding to definitive planning and preparations for crown and bridge work.

Throughout this book the importance of good plaque control is stressed. In some instances it is advantageous to institute a probationary period in which the patient can demonstrate an understanding of plaque-control procedures and an ability to carry them out routinely. The recording and explaining of plaque and periodontal indices may help the patient to maintain the necessary high standard of plaque control.

Gingivitis or periodontitis, if present, should be dealt with before major restorative procedures are undertaken. Quite apart from the need to ensure that time, and probably money, is not wasted because of unhealthy periodontal tissues, there is the possibility that the level of the gingival margin may be altered following efficient plaque control, and especially if surgery has been undertaken. In some instances it may be helpful to undertake basic tooth preparation and provide temporary or intermediate crowns or bridges, properly contoured and fitting well at the gingival margins. This allows time for the periodontal tissues to heal before the final tooth preparations are undertaken. The relationship between periodontal status and restorative treatment is discussed in Chapter 2.

Caries control is important in two respects. Firstly, if untreated caries remains in the mouth, the oral environment is altered and the liability to caries in other teeth is increased. Secondly, it is important to discover the extent of caries in any tooth because it may affect the outline of a preparation and because of its potential effects on the pulp. In teeth with deep carious lesions, it may be necessary to maintain them with temporary dressings while waiting to discover whether or not the pulp retains full vitality. If there is doubt about vitality it is generally preferable to undertake elective endodontics rather than risk being forced to do root canal treatment after restorations have been placed. Any teeth in which root canal treatment has been undertaken should be reviewed to ensure that healing has occurred before embarking on tooth preparation.

One other aspect that may require stabilization is the occlusion. Most patients have an occlusal pattern that is satisfactory, even if not ideal, but it should always be assessed and any problems such as deflective contacts remedied. Occlusal considerations are dealt with in Chapter 3. The patient should be given an adequate time to adjusst to any changes made before bridge work is started.

Treatment of caries in inlay, crown and bridge work

The final outline of an inlay cavity depends on the extent of the carious lesion. Where this is minimal, penetration is made into dentine and the cavity is extended to the classic outline. This is determined by the class of cavity, the tooth form and the need to remove adjacent areas on the tooth surface. With widespread destruction by caries, the undermined enamel must be removed and the carious dentine at the amelodentine junction excavated. However, the outline of the cavity is only decided provisionally because subsequent modification may be necessary.

In crown preparation, extensive caries should be removed in the usual manner and the resulting cavity made retentive before filling with glass ionomer, amalgam or composite resin (Figure 1.4). Such a material may then be treated as sound tooth substance during the rest of the procedure, but the periphery of the preparation should be tttaken at least 1 mm beyond its limit. Retentive grooves, if required, should be placed in sound tooth substance. In bridge work, caries of the abutment teeth is treated in the same manner as in individual crowns.

Retention and resistance

Conventional restorations

There are basic principles that govern the shaping of a cavity to ensure a cast restoration is retained securely and remains stable in the cavity. A consideration of these principles, before embarking on tooth preparation, will avoid many failures.

The restoration should have only one path of insertion so that it is forced to slide along tooth surfaces and strong frictional forces would have to be overcome to displace it. At least two walls of the preparation must oppose

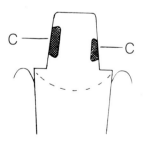
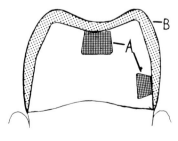

Figure 1.4 Undercuts formed by the removal of caries or old restorations during crown preparation may be eliminated with glass ionomer cement (C) or amalgam (A) before completion of the preparation for a gold veneer crown (B)

each other to provide retention in the line of insertion. If the restoration is to resist the forces that tend to displace it from the tooth, the preparation must be designed to provide this resistance. These features of retention and resistance merit more detailed discussion.

Retention

It is convenient to divide retention into three types:

1. Intracoronal retention uses internal tooth walls facing each other, as is the case with inlays.
2. Extracoronal retention uses external tooth walls opposing each other, as is the case for most crowns.
3. Accessory retention is used where insufficient tooth substance is available under types 1 and 2. Additional opposing surfaces can be made by sinking slots, posts or pins into the dentine. Although particularly valuable as additional retention, pins and intraradicular posts can also be used as the sole means of retention.

The best possible arrangement would be parallel walls, but attempts to cut a preparation with parallel walls may result in undetected undercuts. The walls are therefore made to diverge slightly for intracoronal retention and converge slightly for extracoronal retention. An angle of taper greater than 5° affects retention and this ideally should be regarded as the limit in teeth with short clinical crowns (Figure 1.5).

These principles are easy to apply when there is plenty of tooth to support the preparation, but the shape of the tooth may make it difficult to gain sufficient retention. The haphazard removal of tooth substance during the preparation for a full veneer crown on even a substantial tooth such as an upper molar can lead to a loss of optimum retention. Furthermore the entire length of the longest side of a tooth cannot necessarily be used for retention unless it can be provided with an opposing side.

It is a good principle to consider habitually the retention of any preparation separately from the removal of tooth substance for other purposes.

Resistance

Opposing walls will only 'retain' if other aspects of the design prevent the restoration from moving out of contact with the walls. There is little difficulty in realizing that any number of parallel sides are useless if the part of the tooth which they enclose is so weak as to break off under the stress of

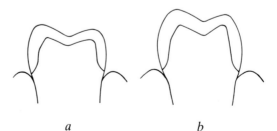

Figure 1.5 (a) Near parallelism is important to gain retention with a short clinical crown. (b) With longer opposing walls the preparation will be sufficiently retentive with slightly greater convergence

a   *b*

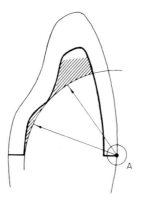

Figure 1.6 If the shaded areas are removed during preparation, retention will be lost between labial and palatal surfaces and the crown will tend to rotate around point A

mastication. The shape of the natural crown may also affect this resistance form of the preparation. For instance, the principles of retention of a jacket crown preparation for an upper central incisor can be satisfied using only the mesial and distal walls, yet the cingulum wall and the length of the preparation are critical in preventing the crown from being displaced from the tooth (Figure 1.6).

The occlusal part of a two-surface gold inlay must be in the form of a dovetail to prevent the approximal displacement. The walls of the lock must also be deep enough to prevent rotation out of the cavity. If, for reasons of appearance, the buccal surface is not available for use as an opposing wall, slots are used on the proximal opposing walls, as in the case of partial veneer crowns.

Pins

Pins may be used as accessory retention but there is the practical difficulty of aligning multiple pins. The taper of the walls within a pinhole is determined by the bur used to cut it. Wrought-wire pins with parallel sides fit holes cut with a twist drill and provide good retention. Cast pins can be made to holes cut with tapered fissure burs and although the retention they provide is not quite so good, there is more latitude when several pinholes are prepared.

The use of a pin is an excellent method of gaining additional retention when only a small amount of dentine is available. Used as accessory retention in an inlay preparation the pin can take the place of a missing axial wall or can provide the locking action that will prevent displacement. Even when the clinical crown of the tooth has been destroyed, it can be rebuilt as an amalgam core retained by multiple pins, as described in Chapter 8.

On occasion, pins may be used as the sole means of retention, as in the pinledge restoration. Experience has shown, however, that this type of restoration is prone to failure because of cement fracture and leakage.

Careful consideration must be given to where pins are to be placed, how many are used and what should be their length, diameter and material. The potential sites are limited because pins must be placed entirely in dentine where they will not involve the pulp or the periodontium. If the gold connecting the pins is regarded as a bar that does not contribute to retention, the gold would tend to rotate around only one pin and be subject to bending stresses. This would also happen about the line drawn between two pins. A third pin added to make a triangle will form the minimal stable system when pins alone are used.

Pins should be as thick as possible to resist torsional stresses, but it is unlikely that room can be found for anything larger than 0.75 mm in diameter. Iridio–platinum pins of less than 0.5 mm in diameter are probably too easily bent. Pins should be as long as possible, but it is doubtful whether the difficulties of siting multiple pins more than 3 mm into dentine is worthwhile. Should it prove impossible to place pins longer than 2 mm, their number can be increased above the minimum of three.

The metal joining the pins must be strong enough to resist distortion or the restoration will leak and fail. When the amount of dentine is sufficient, strength may be gained by grooving the preparation between the pinholes so that a 'girder' is formed between the pins in the resultant casting.

Adhesive restorations

Adhesive restorations rely upon micro-mechanical or chemical bonding to tooth tissue. They frequently cover only a single surface of a tooth, so considerations of retention and resistance applicable to conventional restorations cannot apply to them.

Retention is largely dependent on gaining the maximum possible bonding area and meticulous attention to detail when bonding. Shear stress in occlusion should be minimized and cingulum or occlusal rests provided wherever possible.

Additional retention may be gained by the preparation of shallow grooves or boxes and, in posterior preparations, a 'wrap-round' design can be used to increase the enamel bonding area. This can also provide increased stability because tooth walls can oppose each other mesially and distally.

Types of restoration

1. Intracoronal. For example, inlays.
2. Adhesive veneer.
3. Partial veneer crown. These have a veneer of metal covering from three-quarters to seven-eighths of the clinical crown.
4. Full crown.
   (a) Full veneer crown.
   (b) Metal–ceramic crown.
   (c) Porcelain jacket crown. These are usually restricted to anterior teeth.
5. Post-retained crown. These are normally made as a separate jacket cemented to a post-retained core.

Full versus partial coverage

Although sufficient clinical crown must be present to retain an artificial crown, full coverage can provide strength and protection by embracing remaining tooth structure with a covering of tough material over the whole surface.

Jacket and veneer crowns provide this full coverage of the prepared clinical crown of a tooth. Good retention is possible because near parallel walls can be prepared on the axial walls and because of the relatively large surface area available. Resistance to lateral displacement is also excellent. It may be impossible to remove sufficient tooth substance from the labial surface to accommodate a facing without endangering the pulp. This should be assessed early in treatment planning and the alternative of a partial veneer crown considered. To make the discovery during the preparation casts doubt on the operator's foresight.

The partial veneer crown preparation requires the removal of less tooth substance than a full-coverage crown. It maintains the appearance of the natural tooth by retaining the labial or buccal enamel and preserves the natural contour and may therefore be preferred to a full metal crown. For these reasons a partial veneer crown is frequently used as a bridge retainer when the abutment tooth has a sound, or almost sound, clinical crown.

An adhesive (minimal preparation) retainer is even more conservative than a partial veneer crown and may be preferred in many lightly-stressed situations.

Design of gingival margins

However perfectly the gingival margin of a preparation is finished and however excellently the restoration is polished and adapted to the tooth, there is some detrimental effect on the gingivae. Plaque cannot be removed as readily from the junction between restorations and tooth as it can from a tooth surface. It is, therefore, advocated that the gingival margins of restorations should normally be placed just supragingivally where the patient can keep them clean (Figure 1.7). The margins should, if possible, follow the natural gingival contour.

Where caries has extended to a level below the soft tissues, it is often possible to re-create a supragingival margin by the judicious removal of soft tissue, either with scalpel or using electrosurgery, but these procedures should be undertaken with care, and in some instances subgingival margins may have to be accepted.

Where appearance is important, such as the labial aspects of porcelain crowns in the anterior part of the mouth, the margins should normally be placed within the gingival sulcus. Where very short clinical crowns exist, it may be advisable to extend the preparation subgingivally in order to gain additional retention for the restoration.

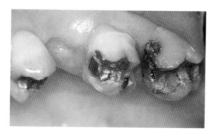

Figure 1.7 Supragingival finishing line on crown preparation for an upper first molar

Figure 1.8 The shaded area represents the saving of tooth substance if a shoulderless preparation (dotted line) is used instead of a shoulder with a bevel (continuous line)

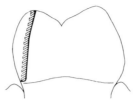

In all instances it is necessary for the treatment plan to consider the management of soft tissues as well as hard tissues, and to ensure that gingivae are healthy before tooth preparation is undertaken. This is especially important where anterior crowns are to be undertaken in order to avoid the margins of the crowns becoming visible.

Shoulder versus shoulderless preparations

Whether or not a crown preparation needs a shoulder depends mainly on the bulk of crown material required, which in turn is determined by its inherent strength. A shoulderless preparation is preferable whenever gold is used because the preparation is easier and less tooth substance is removed, which means that damage to the pulp is reduced. The saving of tooth substance is clearly seen in Figure 1.8 in which a shoulderless preparation is superimposed on a preparation with a shoulder.

To avoid a ragged finish to a crown constructed on a shoulderless preparation, it is essential to have a clearly defined margin to which the wax pattern can be finished. A cavo-surface angle of approximately 135° achieved by a full chamfer as shown in Figure 1.9a and 1.9b, is therefore recommended because it provides a clearly defined margin with minimal removal of tissue. A smaller cavo-surface angle would expose a greater thickness of cement at the margin (Figure 1.9c). A larger angle results in poor definition of the margin and provides an indistinguishable finishing line for the technician to work to (Figure 1.9d).

It is necessary to create a slip joint rather than a butt joint in order to minimize the inevitable gap between casting and preparation.

It is apparent that the cervical gap is smaller than the occlusal gap when

Figure 1.9 Types of cervical finishing lines. (a) 135° cavo-surface angle. (b) Shoulder with bevel, achieving 135° cavo-surface angle. (c) Shoulder without bevel: cavo-surface angle 90°. (d) 180° cavo-surface angle

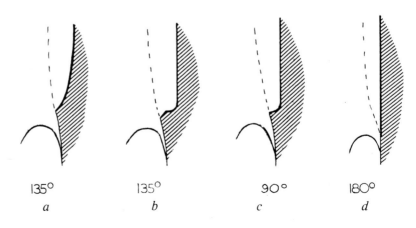

135°   135°   90°   180°
a   b   c   d

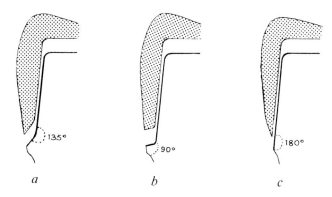

135°   90°   180°

a   *b*   *c*

Figure 1.10 The gap at the cervical margin for a cavo-surface angle of 135° is less than the gap at the occlusal surface. For a 90° angle it is the same dimension as the axial gap. (After Fusayama)

the cavo-surface angle is 135°, but is as large as the occlusal gap when the cavo-surface angle is 90°. There is, however, no relationship between the occlusal and cervical gaps when the cavo-surface angle is 180° (Figure 1.10). The relationship between the occlusal and cervical gaps can be expressed mathematically.

There are three indications for the preparation of a shoulder:

1. When an all-porcelain crown is to be made.
2. When a metal crown is to be faced with porcelain.
3. If caries or cervical abrasion has already made a step unavoidable at the gingival margin.

An even thickness of porcelain is essential for an all-porcelain crown and the shoulder should be prepared to a uniform width. Ideally, this should be 1 mm and because porcelain lacks toughness a butt joint must be made between the material and tooth substance. The cavo-surface angle will therefore be 90° (Figure 1.9a).

A bonded porcelain crown is difficult to construct unless 1.5 mm of space is provided wherever both metal and porcelain have to be accommodated. Elsewhere on the tooth the usual veneer preparation is sufficient. For this type of crown a cavo-surface angle of 135° should be prepared.

The 180° cavo-surface angle (Figure 1.9c) should be avoided whenever possible.

Availability of skilled technical facilities

The knowledge of inlay, crown and bridge construction is useless without the practical means for applying that knowledge both at the chairside and in the laboratory.

It is usual to rely on a technician to construct restorations and every operator needs good technical facilities. Whilst it is an advantage to have a technician on the surgery premises, it is not essential provided that there is an understanding of the techniques used by the operator.

This understanding between a dentist and technician is something that can only be built up over a long period of cooperation, and it is important that the operator tackles nothing beyond the skill of the technician. It is suggested that the dentist embarking on advanced restorative procedures or changing technicians should first reach complete accord on simple restorations before progressing to more complex procedures.

It is essential that instructions to the technician about the design of each restoration or component are clear and complete. This includes any special notes about shape, colour, amount of gold visible and other details, such as where the gold–porcelain junction should be placed in metal–ceramic work.

Chapter 2

Periodontal considerations

However well-made inlays, crowns and bridges may be, the restorations will fail if the teeth do not have sound supporting tissues. An understanding of the interrelationships between soft and hard tissues is, therefore, important.

The clinical gingival sulcus depth normally measures 1–3 mm in health whereas both the epithelial attachment and connective tissue are approximately 1 mm long. Therefore, the alveolar crest is located approximately 2 mm apical to the base of the sulcus (Figure 2.1). Early recognition is a decisive factor in the prevention of progress of periodontal disease. Gingival redness, swelling, and bleeding should be noted and demonstrated to the patient. Many patients suffer from periodontal disease of varying extent for many years without being aware of it. Once they have had their periodontal health restored by education (oral hygiene instruction) and treatment, they are more aware of the early signs of disease, such as bleeding areas.

Margins of restorations should be supragingival if possible and should always end above the epithelial attachment. Unfortunately subgingival margins often extend beyond the gingival sulcus into the junctional epithelium and connective tissues. This causes marginal gingivitis, which may progress to periodontitis resulting in recession, pocketing, or both

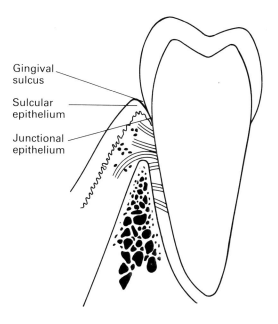

Gingival sulcus

Sulcular epithelium

Junctional epithelium

Figure 2.1 The relationship between the gingival sulcus, the epithelial attachment and the crown of the tooth

Figure 2.2 Ill-fitting subgingival margins on 1|12 retainers causing gingival inflammation

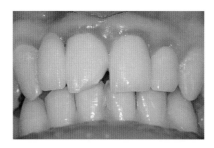

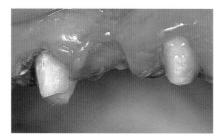

Figure 2.3 Inflammatory response beneath a poorly contoured bridge

(Figures 2.2, 2.3, 2.4). Excessive sulcus depth is characteristic of pocketing and periodontal disease.

Successful long-term restorative dentistry depends upon a healthy periodontium around the tooth being restored. Ideally restorative procedures should not be undertaken in the presence of disease. It is much easier to make precise preparations and obtain accurate impressions where the gingiva is healthy than when it is inflamed and haemorrhagic. All subgingivally placed margins of dental restorations are associated with pathological alteration of the adjacent gingivae. Margins that have already been placed subgingivally may require surgical removal of the overlying soft tissue. The need for subgingival extension of margins to enhance retention may often be overcome by pin techniques or modern adhesive techniques.

When prepparations have to be extended subgingivally because of caries or failed restorations this extension should be limited to the minimum dictated by the conditions. Well-fitted supragingival margins are of no periodontal significance and those placed at the gingival margin result in only an insignificant incidence of gingivitis.

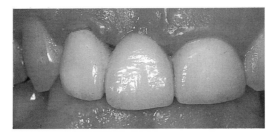

Figure 2.4 Recession at the gingival margin of 2|, which is an ill-fitting bridge retainer

Reasons for subgingival placement of margins:

1. Removal of caries or replacement of faulty restorations.
2. Obtaining adequate retention form for restorations.
3. Prevention or elimination of root sensitivity.
4. Improving appearance.

The margins of tooth preparations should be placed in the regions that are accessible to cleaning by the patient. When subgingival placement is essential for aesthetic reasons, they should be extended only 0.5 mm into the gingival sulcus and should be at least 0.5 mm away from the connective tissue attachment. In fixed prosthodontics, aesthetic reasons may dictate subgingival placement of metal ceramic crown margins especially in the upper anterior region. Only that part of the margin which is visible during normal lip movement is placed subgingivally. The margins on the lingual side are placed supragingivally.

To prepare a tooth for a subgingival margin a minimum of 1.5 to 2.0 mm clinical sulcus depth is required to prevent damage to the epithelial attachment. If the crevice depth is less than 0.5 mm, then the patient and dentist must accept supragingival margins. Immediately following periodontal surgery the dentist is often faced with a crevice less than this depth. Therefore restorative treatment must be delayed until the full new crevice depth develops. In the case of extensive periodontal surgery 2–3 months or more are required for healing. Even when surgery is not required in instances of severe gingival inflammation it takes a month or more after scaling and instruction in oral hygiene before healing is complete.

Temporary restorations and crowns

Any temporary restoration extending subgingivally is a source of gingival irritation just as much as a permanent restoration. Only temporary restorations needed for plaque control and protection against caries should be placed before the hygiene phase. Rough surfaces and poorly fitting margins of temporary restorations will enhance plaque accumulation and gingival irritation. Gingival recession around temporary crowns is minimized by careful tooth preparation, by establishing well-fitting margins and by making the contours of the temporary restoration resemble those of the natural tooth to allow effective plaque control.

Gingival retraction and impressions

If the margin lies at or below the gum, it is necessary to retract or displace the gum temporarily to allow the impression material to record the tooth surface contour apical to the preparation. All retraction methods induce transient trauma to the junction epithelium and connective tissue of the gingival sulcus. If the retraction cord is placed atraumatically against the clean tooth surface in the presence of a healthy periodontium, healing is rapid and uneventful. These cords are available in different widths and stiffness. They may be impregnated with haemostatic or astringent chemicals or be unmedicated.

Electrosurgery

Various electrosurgical techniques have been advocated to facilitate impression-taking. The use of electrosurgical (radiosurgical) units results in cellular healing comparable to a scalpel wound. Controlled depth cutting electrode tips avoid bone trauma but injure gingival fibres if the tip is not angled properly in the sulcus. Electrosurgery allows the removal of excess gingival tissue, which impedes access during preparation or adversely affects aesthetics or retention (Figure 2.5a, 2.5b. 2.5c. 2.5d). It may also be used to control gingival bleeding. Electrosurgery should be used as a backup technique rather than a substitute for gingival retraction cord. It may complement gingival retraction when the papillary tissue overhangs the retraction cord interdentally and the electrode tip may be used to thin the tissue without reducing its vertical height. Severe tissue damage can result if the operator uses faulty equipment, inappropriate current setting, poor choice of electrode or incorrect application technique.

Cementation and polishing of restorations

It is much easier to adjust the design and finish of restorations before rather than after they are permanently cemented. Excess cement, which is not completely removed after final cementation, will act as a source of irritation.

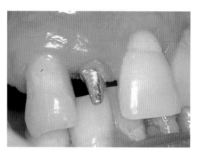

a

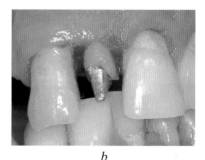

b

Figure 2.5 (a) An unretentive core of a post in 2|. The post had adequate length but could not be removed. (b) The removal of gum from around the 2| allows for a more retentive preparation for a jacket crown. (c) Post-tissue healing and the completed preparation. (d) The fitted crown

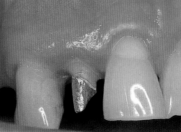

c

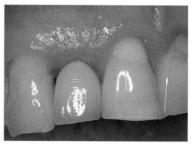

d

Periodontal significance of the design of restorations

The principal cause of periodontal disease is plaque both on teeth and at restoration margins. Overcontouring of restorations is a much greater hazard to health than is undercontour or lack of contour because both supragingival and subgingival plaque accumulation may be increased. A frequent mistake is to make bulging, rounded buccal surfaces on metal ceramic crowns, and the main reason for this is inadequate removal of labial tooth substance during preparation of vital teeth. The technician then has to make an exaggerated contour to create space for both metal and porcelain. Interproximal overcontouring of restorations is more common than buccolingual overcontouring. The proximal surfaces of natural teeth gingival to the contact areas are either flat or concave. In patients in whom the interproximal surfaces of anterior teeth are not occluded with gingival papillae, as is often seen after periodontal surgery, there is a common tendency to make artificial crowns too wide mesiodistally towards the gingival margin in order to close the open spaces. This produces unaesthetic restorations and gingival irritation. The result is a deeper than normal col, and hyperplastic buccal and lingual papillae between posterior teeth. A larger than normal interproximal space is not a periodontal handicap because the proximal surfaces are readily accessible to plaque control.

In the furcation region of teeth, attention must be paid to the preparation and the contours of the crown. A concave dip in the preparation and the marginal aspect of the crown should be made to correspond to the exposed furcation (Figure 2.6). Restorations are often poorly finished in furcation regions and those having overhanging or thick margins make this a vulnerable location.

Interproximal contacts

Open contacts without food impaction are of no periodontal significance and they should not be filled up with dental restorations if the occlusion is stable and the teeth are intact. The function of the interproximal contact is to prevent both vertical and horizontal food impaction.

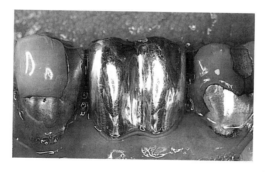

Figure 2.6 The vertical groove in the mid-buccal surface makes plaque removal from the bifurcation region easier

Embrasure spaces

These should be sufficiently open to allow easy access for interproximal brushes, floss threaders and other interdental plaque removal devices.

Crown lengthening procedures

These may be required where there is excess gum, or to expose preparation margins or where there is extensive caries close to the alveolar crest or tooth fracture apical to the epithelial attachment. Crown lengthening may also be indicated in cases where there is insufficient clinical crown length for adequate retention of restorations.

The rationale for crown lengthening is to gain more vertical length for crown retention whilst allowing a 3–4 mm distance to be maintained between the crown margin and the alveolar crest in order to preserve periodontal health. The root morphology, tooth position, alveolar support and the overall strategic value of the tooth/teeth should be assessed pre-operatively. Crown lengthening procedures are usually accomplished by apically repositioned flaps and osseous surgery.

Osseous recontouring is blended with the adjacent alveolar crest to produce an even contour. Flap margins are sutured at or just above the new alveolar crest and sufficient time must be allowed for healing before proceeding with restorative treatment. Occasionally the orthodontic technique of 'forced tooth eruption' may be used to lengthen the clinical crown of fractured teeth. Crown lengthening may be a major surgical procedure and, can result in furcation involvement and severe postoperative root sensitivity. Patient selection should therefore be highly discriminating in this respect.

Plaque control and maintenance

Inlays, crowns and bridges must be designed and contoured to help plaque control. The patient must be educated and motivated to maintain a good oral hygiene. Methods of plaque control should always be tailored to the individual needs and ability. Suitable mirrors and plaque disclosing agents are always helpful.

The patient must be shown correct tooth brushing techniques and a choice

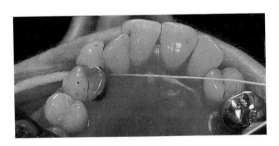

Figure 2.7 Removal of plaque from the tissue surface of the pontic with superfloss. The nylon lead filament helps in threading the floss through the embrasures

of brushes. Interdental plaque removal aids, such as dental tape, floss, interdental brushes, floss threaders and super floss, are all helpful in the removal of plaque from teeth, bridges and splints (Figure 2.7).

Sequence of treatment

The sequence of treatment for a patient requiring periodontal care as part of an overall programme of restorative treatment may be summarized as follows.

Periodontal examination noting:

1. Areas of bleeding on probing.
2. Pocket depths.
3. Overcontoured or ill-fitting restorations.

Initial treatment may include:

1. Patient motivation, education and instruction in plaque control.
2. Scaling and polishing.
3. Elimination of plaque retention factors (removal of overhangs, replacement of overcontoured/ill-fitting restorations.

The next phase of treatment:

1. Reassessment, continued plaque control and monitoring.
2. Root planing.

The patient may now be ready for surgical periodontal treatment. A waiting period for healing may then be required before proceeding to inlay, crown and bridge work.

Chapter 3

Occlusal considerations

Occlusion is the contact of the maxillary and mandibular teeth on closure (a static position). Articulation, however, refers to the mandible in motion, a dynamic relation. An understanding of the importance of all the components of the masticatory system in normal function, parafunction and dysfunction is important for the restorative dentist. The restoration of teeth by inlays, crowns and bridges provides an opportunity not only for repairing lost tooth tissue but also for obtaining a functional occlusal surface where this is lacking due to maleruption, tilting or loss of teeth. Open contact points can be closed, marginal ridges made level and unopposed teeth stabilized in the arch. Where an unopposed tooth has overerupted, it can be reshaped to align with the arch and a new occlusal surface can be provided by means of an inlay, onlay or crown.

Few topics in dentistry generate as much controversy or conflict as occlusion. The dentist should recognize that a wide range of normal exists when determining the appropriateness of occlusal treatment. The possibility of a patient with a symptom-free 'adapting occlusion' developing occlusal disharmony as a result of restorative treatment may increase with the number and complexity of the restorations. The level of adaptive tolerance varies between individuals and, over a period of time, within the same individual. When planning a restoration involving the occlusal surface of a tooth one must know how to direct the occlusal forces favourably through the tooth (and the restorative material). The rationale for occlusal treatment is to preserve, restore, and maintain the state of normal function. This state exists when there is harmony between the occlusal morphology and neuromuscular function within the adaptive range (an adapting occlusion). Exceeding the patient's capacity to adapt commonly results in occlusal disharmony. Every restoration should be designed to conform to the functional tolerance limits of the patient. Specifically, the occlusion should be tailored to the individual.

Terminology and definitions

A number of definitions is basic to an understanding of the mechanism of occlusion sufficient for the designing and construction of inlays, crowns and bridges.

Intercuspal position (ICP)   The relationship of the mandible to the maxilla where there is maximum intercuspation.

Retruded axis/terminal hinge axis (RA/THA)   On opening, the mandible can hinge about a horizontal axis called the retruded axis, permitting an incisal opening of approximately 2.5 cm with the condyles in the retruded position.

Retruded contact position (RCP)   The relationship of the mandible to the maxilla at which initial occlusal contact has occurred after closure about the retruded axis (posterior and most superior rotary hinge axis). Approximately 90% of individuals have a discrepancy (slide) between the retruded contact position and the intercuspal position (Figure 3.1).

Retruded axis registration (RAR)   A 'tooth apart' interocclusal record used to allow mounting of casts on an articulator (semi-adjustable type) for diagnostic purposes (or occlusal splint fabrication).

Rest position (RP)   When not in function the mandible normally remains in the 'rest position' in which there is 2–4 mm separation between the teeth of the upper and lower jaws.

Vertical dimension of occlusion (VDO)   This is the measurement of the face height when the mandible is in the intercuspal position. The separation between the RP and VDO is termed 'the freeway space' and represents the interocclusal distance.

Anterior guidance (AG)   The effect of the articulating surfaces of the anterior teeth on mandibular movement.

Canine guidance (CG)   An occlusion where only the canines are in contact on the working side during a lateral excursion of the mandible (Figure 3.2).

Group function (GF)   An occlusion where there are two or more pairs of teeth contacting on the working side during a lateral excursion of the mandible (Figure 3.3).

Working side (WS)   The side to which the mandible moves during a lateral excursion.

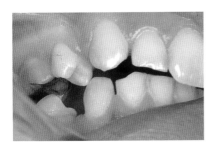

a

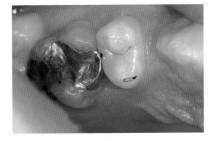

b

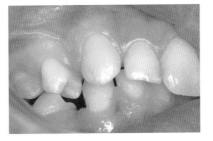

c

Figure 3.1 (a) Retruded contact position. The initial contact on the retruded arc of closure occurs between the distal incline of the $\overline{3|}$ cusp and the mesial aspect of the $\underline{4|}$ palatal cusp. (b) Slide from retruded contact position to intercuspal position is marked on $\underline{4|}$ with articulating paper. (c) Intercuspal position

Figure 3.2 Canine guidance in right lateral excursion

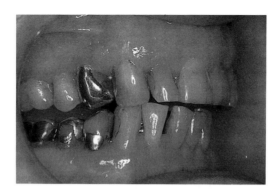

Figure 3.3 Group function occlusion with <u>6543</u>| contacting during lateral excursion

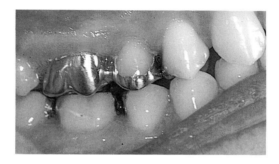

Non-working side (NWS)   The side away from which the mandible moves during a lateral excursion.

Occlusal interference (OI)   Contact between teeth in opposing arches, which deflects the path of mandibular movement and interferes with harmonious jaw function. Occlusal interferences may occur on the working side, non-working side, during a protrusive excursion, or on the retruded arc of closure (a retruded interference).

Parafunctional movement (PM)   These movements of the mandible are not part of mastication and speech. They are usually habitual and include tooth to tooth contacts (bruxism and clenching), tooth to soft tissue contacts (lip biting), soft tissue to soft tissue contacts (abnormal swallowing patterns), and foreign body to tooth contacts (pipe clenching).

Functionally generated pathway (FGP)   Static registration of dynamic mandibular movements.

Occlusal assessment

Careful history taking and clinical examination are important parts of an occlusal examination. Clinical examination alone may not provide adequate information for diagnostic and treatment planning purposes. The patient's complaints about lack of masticatory efficiency, excessive or uneven occlusal wear, limitation of mandibular movement, discomfort or pain on chewing and a sense of occlusal awareness following occlusal adjustment or restoration should all be recorded. Further investigations may be required,

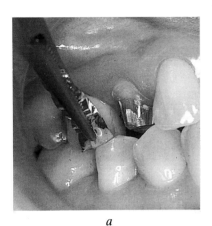 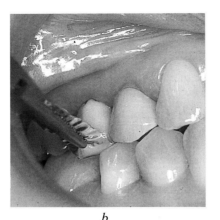

a *b*

Figure 3.4 (a) Shimstock is used to show occlusal contact on teeth adjacent to the prepared upper first premolar. (b) Crown tried in and the contact on teeth is as before

including radiographs, vitality tests and articulated study casts. The examination should be both extra-oral and intra-oral.

The patient's intercuspal position is first examined to determine whether a stable posterior occlusal relationship exists. Axial loading in intercuspal position should be present on several pairs of opposing posterior teeth, sufficient to maintain the vertical dimension of occlusion. The patient's lateral and protrusive occlusal relationships are examined to determine the nature of the lateral guidance (canine guided or group function) and whether there is satisfactory anterior guidance. This should be sufficiently steep to allow posterior teeth to separate during protrusive/lateral excursions but not steep enough to initiate parafunction. Occlusal interferences found during this examination are recorded and then the patient's mandible is guided on the retruded arc of closure to the position of initial tooth contact and the nature and extent of the slide from retruded contact to intercuspal position is assessed.

Signs and symptoms of mandibular dysfunction are noted together with evidence of excessive tooth wear. Increased tooth mobility, fracture of restorations or teeth and symptoms of mandibular dysfunctions may all result from increased muscle activity. Accurate marking of tooth contacts during occlusal examination is important. Thin, non-smearing articulating paper or shimstock can be used to evaluate the degree of occlusal contact (Figure 3.4).

Assessment of stability of the intercuspal position

Posterior occlusal stability may be lost because of extraction and non-replacement of teeth or the placement of restorations with inadequate occlusal contours. The diagnosis of occlusal instability is based on the occurrence of one or more clinical signs and symptoms, such as increased tooth wear; fracture of teeth or loss of restorations; hypermobility and drifting; and mandibular dysfunction.

Sufficient pairs of posterior teeth should contact simultaneously in order to direct occlusal forces axially and stabilize the teeth and the tempero-mandibular joints in intercuspal position. Proximal tooth contacts play an

Figure 3.5 (a and b) Try in of crown 4| showing axial loading with contacts between marginal ridges (a) and opposing cusp tips (b)

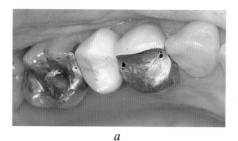

a

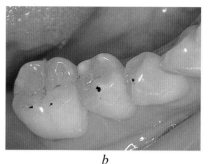

b

important role in maintaining posterior tooth stability, particulary if intercuspal contacts are not ideally placed to achieve axial loading. Axial loading may result from contact either between the tip of a supporting cusp and the opposing fossa or by the occlusion between opposing inclined plane contacts (Figure 3.5). Edentulous spaces may require restoration to prevent drifting and tilting of adjacent teeth. However, posterior occlusal stability may exist despite the loss of teeth. The neuromuscular system can adapt to maintain the intercuspal position despite tooth loss or wear. The patient may develop a habitual path of closure guiding the mandible around and away from occlusal interferences and bring the teeth together in a new intercuspal position. When replacing restorations care should be taken to maintain stable occlusal contacts that conform to the pre-existing intercuspal position.

Occlusal analysis and diagnostic wax-up procedures

Diagnostic study casts mounted on a semi-adjustable articulator permit an analysis of the occlusion in isolation from the influence of the patient's neuromuscular system. Occlusal interferences in the retruded arc of closure may be identified and alterations to the occlusal surfaces of the teeth on the casts may be made in order to identify appropriate treatment. This may include trial occlusal adjustment and diagnostic waxing to allow the dentist to find out in advance the extent of the occlusal alteration required. For example when a posterior bridge is planned and one of the proposed abutments makes initial contact on the retruded arc of closure then failure to diagnose and treat this pre-operatively, may lead to fracture of provisional restorations or occlusal perforation of the retainer during adjustment at the fit stage. Occlusal reduction during tooth preparation may be compromised by mandibular repositioning and a change in the intercuspal position brought about by elimination of the retruded contact during crown preparation.

Diagnostic use of provisional restorations

Satisfactory coronal contours for anterior tooth restorations are required for appearance, speech and anterior guidance. When several anterior teeth

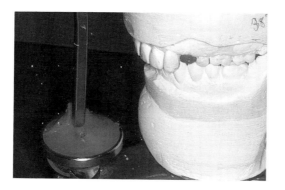

Figure 3.6 A custom acrylic anterior guide table

have been prepared it is important to provide the technician with adequate information to allow correct shaping of coronal tooth contours. Otherwise the appearance and function of the restorations will be arbitrarily determined by the technician and the result may be unsatisfactory.

If the anterior guidance was satisfactory pre-operatively, the technician may copy the incisal edge length and palatal contours of the unprepared teeth in the final restorations by waxing up against a palatal stone or resin index made on the pre-operative study cast and fitted to the working cast. The same technique may be employed to copy contours of provisional restorations that are deemed to be satisfactory after trial wear and adjustment.

Alternatively, casts of the adjusted provisional restorations may be mounted on a semi-adjustable articulator in order to allow a custom acrylic anterior guide table to be created (Figure 3.6). This will allow the technician to copy the anterior guidance that has been developed and verified as satisfactory intra-orally. The incisal edges of the lower anterior teeth articulating against the palatal contours of the upper anterior teeth in excursive movements provide the anterior guidance.

Occlusal adjustment

Indications for occlusal adjustment include:

1. Occlusal interferences associated with increased tooth mobility, drifting, failure of restorations, pain or discomfort.
2. Occlusal interferences that involve the teeth to be restored.

When undertaking an occlusal analysis it is necessary to decide whether occlusal adjustment is required before restorative treatment can begin. When few restorations are needed, and the teeth to be restored do not provide the RCP contact, the posterior occlusion is stable and there is no evidence of mandibular dysfunction, then occlusal adjustment should not be required. Many of the occlusal problems encountered when making restorations to conform to the existing intercuspal position are due to uneven opposing occlusal surfaces and/or lack of adequate anterior guidance (Figure 3.7).

It is usually necessary to carry out occlusal adjustment before proceeding

Figure 3.7 (a) A patient with missing 65| and overerupted $\overline{6}$| before bridge work. This is a potential occlusal problem. (b) After treatment. The $\overline{6}$| required reduction and crowning to establish a satisfactory occlusal plane before restoring the upper space with a bridge

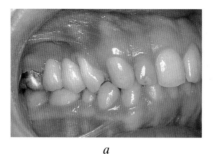
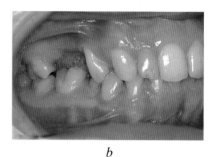

a   *b*

with tooth preparation and restoration. Failure to do so may lead to early failure of restorations.

Use of articulators

Articulators are mechanical devices that allow information to be transferred from the mouth to the laboratory about the way in which the mandibular and the maxillary teeth occlude. If the dentist's only concern is about the relationship of the opposing teeth in the position of maximal intercuspation then the design and use of the articulator is greatly simplified. Since this is a static position, the articulator would only need to act as a rigid hinge. The mandible, however, does not act as a simple hinge, rather it is capable of rotation about axes in three planes. The occlusal morphology of any restoration must accommodate the free passage of the opposing teeth without interfering with mandibular movement.

Articulators may be classified into four main categories:

1. Simple hinge.
2. Average value.
3. Semi-adjustable.
4. Fully adjustable.

This classification is based on the ability of the instruments to copy mandibular movements. No existing articulator will reproduce all mandibular movements precisely, which is also not their primary objective. The aim should be to make a restoration with an occlusal morphology compatible with mandibular movement. The choice of an articulator will depend upon the clinical situation and the knowledge and ability of the operator. This choice should be based on a sound knowledge of the advantages and disadvantages of each type.

Simple hinge articulators and cast relators (class I)
Simple 'barn door' hinge articulators consist of two rigid arms united by a hinge and they may have a set screw adjustment posteriorly to act as a vertical stop (Figure 3.8a). They permit hinge opening only around a horizontal axis whose distance from the cast is determined arbitrarily. Since the distance between the teeth and the axis of rotation is much shorter than in the mouth these intruments may produce significant occlusal errors. They should be reserved for observing static intercuspal relationships or for the

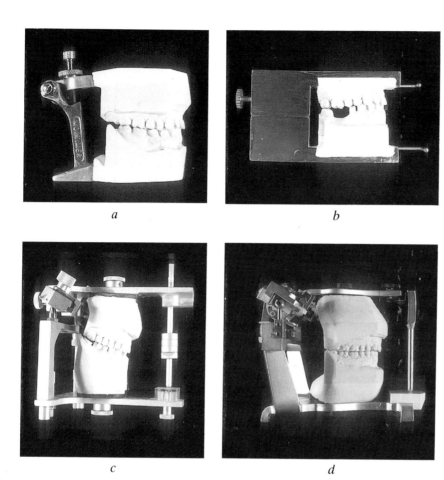

a   *b*

c   *d*

Figure 3.8 (a) Hinge articulator. (b) Jelenko cast relator. (c) Semi-adjustable articulator (Whip-Mix). (d) Fully adjustable articulator (Denar)

construction of single crowns conforming to the existing intercuspal position. The restoration should not be required to contact intra-orally in any position other than the intercuspal position. Restorations made on this type of instrument may require adjustment in the mouth to remove protrusive and lateral interferences, particularly when the anterior guidance is shallow.

Cast relators, such as the Jelenko Verticulator (Figure 3.8b), are used in the same situation as the hinge articulator but they are capable of more precise cast location. The upper member of the articulator moves up and down on a metal post or posts enabling the cast or casts to be brought into precise intercuspal contact.

Average value articulator (class II)
These instruments are capable of lateral and protrusive movements. However, the relationship between the intercondylar axis on the instrument and on the cast is arbitrarily determined. They are incapable of reproducing mandibular movements accurately. The angles at which the condyles move are fixed according to 'average values'. These instruments offer little advantage over simple hinge articulators or hand-held casts in the construction of single units.

Semi-adjustable articulators (class III)

These instruments are generally suitable for the examination of casts as part of an occlusal assessment and for the construction of most crowns and bridges. They are designed to be of an anatomical size in order to minimize discrepancies in tooth/hinge axis radius and intercondylar distance. They are used with a facebow record, which allows the relationship between the retruded axis and the teeth to be transferred from the patient to the articulator. In addition, it is possible to adjust the angle of condylar movements both in the sagittal and horizontal planes.

Semi-adjustable articulators allow an approximate simulation of lateral and protrusive mandibular movements. The radius of movement on the articulator closely reproduces that on the arc of tooth closure. They will reproduce the direction and end-point but not the intermediate track of the tooth movements. Semi-adjustable articulators may have their 'condyles' on the lower member and the 'fossae' on the upper member or vice versa. The former type is preferred and the ability to remove the upper member of the articulator is a great help to the technician when waxing up restorations (Figure 3.8c). Semi-adjustable articulators are helpful when multiple restorations or several fixed bridges are being made.

Semi-adjustable articulators may be employed successfully even in complex cases provided the procedure is broken down into a number of manageable stages as follows:

1. Stabilization of the posterior occlusion.
2. Establishment of satisfactory anterior guidance.
3. Restoration of the anterior teeth.
4. Restoration of the posterior teeth.

Fully adjustable articulators (class IV)

The final step in the progression of articulators has been the development of the fully adjustable instrument (Figure 3.8d). These may be calibrated to duplicate the border movements of the mandible to a high degree of accuracy. While these instruments are most valuable in restoring complex cases where there is minimal anterior guidance or group function exists, they are expensive and their use requires a high degree of expertise and time.

Occlusal registration for restoration

Occlusal records may be divided into tooth apart and tooth together (contacting) records. The former type are used for diagnostic purposes and the latter for restoration. Retruded axis registration is a tooth apart inter-occlusal record used to allow the mounting of casts on a semi-adjustable articulator for diagnostic purposes or for making occlusal splints.

Inter-occlusal registrations are accomplished with various materials and techniques. Materials should initially be fluid to avoid displacing the teeth or mandible during closure. They should record the incisal/occlusal surfaces of the teeth accurately, and should set rigid, providing a definite seat or location into which the casts may be placed. They should also be easy to manipulate, and dimensionally accurate on setting and storage.

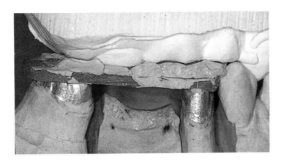

Figure 3.9 Zinc oxide eugenol paste record of the intercuspal position made using a resin base support

Waxes

Wax is widely accepted as an inter-occlusal recording material because it is easy to use. Wax inter-occlusal records are, however, generally inaccurate, unstable, and inconsistent because of their thermoplastic nature and dimensional instability.

When wax is used, a hard variety is preferred (Moyco extra hard) and it should be evenly softened in a water-bath before use. It may be relined with zinc oxide eugenol paste to establish a final accurate inter-occlusal record. Casts should be transferred to the articulator as soon as possible when wax records are used.

Zinc oxide eugenol pastes

Zinc oxide eugenol paste is an effective inter-occlusal registration material and its advantages include fluidity before setting and dimensional stability after setting. It is brittle in thin section and therefore may require a resin platform or base support (Figure 3.9).

Plaster of Paris

Records of impressions in plaster are accurate, rigid after setting, and do not distort on storage. However, the material is difficult to handle intra-orally because of its very fluid nature and its susceptibility to moisture during setting. The final record is also brittle in thin section.

Polymeric impression materials

A number of additional silicones and polyether materials are used for inter-occlusal registration. These materials are accurate, dimensionally stable after setting, exhibit minimal resistance to mandibular closure and do not require a carrier vehicle. However, they are resilient upon setting and inaccuracies may result from distortion during cast mounting. These records are trimmed to remove all excess material and only the cusp tip indentations are preserved.

Acrylic resins

The most frequent application of acrylic resin for inter-occlusal records is for the fabrication of simple intercuspal 'stop' records. Acrylic resin (Duralay) copings made by direct or indirect techniques allow stabilization of the mandible in the intercuspal position following preparation of teeth. When multiple posterior teeth have been prepared or when a space exists between teeth (for example, when a bridge is made), then an acrylic platform is made to serve as a vehicle for a more fluid and accurate recording, such as impression plaster or zinc oxide eugenol paste.

The anatomic index or core

If the existing occlusal surface of the tooth to be restored is satisfactory, or can be made so, then an index should be made of this and related to the working cast by means of a cast relator (see Figure 3.8b) to allow the existing occlusal morphology to be copied in the wax pattern. This type of index is known as an anatomical index. If the existing occlusal surface is not satisfactory then an anatomic index may still be used provided it is made of a correctly adjusted provisional restoration.

Such an index is easily and quickly made with an FGP tray and quick setting artificial stone. It is important to include as many teeth as possible in the quadrant to ensure good stability of the tray. If the tooth or teeth to be restored have other teeth anteriorly and posteriorly then stability of the tray is ensured. With a posterior tooth, the occlusion of four or more teeth anterior to it will similarly ensure tray stability. The technician will be able to reproduce the original occlusal anatomy in the restorations using the anatomic index and the master cast. No occlusal registration or opposing cast are required.

Functionally generated pathway technique

A simple but very effective method for recording all the pathways traced by the movements of the opposing teeth was developed by Meyer in the early 1930s. In this technique soft 'functional' wax is placed over the occlusal surface of the prepared tooth or teeth and the patient is guided through various excursions. The opposing teeth chew the wax away until the remaining teeth in the arches occlude normally. Excess wax overlying the marginal ridges of the adjacent teeth is removed and impression plaster is built up over the wax and extended to cover the adjacent teeth. The tooth to be prepared should have unprepared teeth anterior and posterior to it, in order to allow accurate seating of the functional core on the working cast. The involved teeth should be immobile. Occlusal interferences are eliminated before this method is used and opposing teeth must have satisfactory occlusal contours. The technique is best used in the restoration of upper posterior teeth where the posterior occlusion and anterior guidance are satisfactory (Figure 3.10).

Table 3.1 summarizes the types of occlusal record and articulators indicated for specific situations.

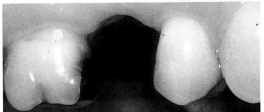

a

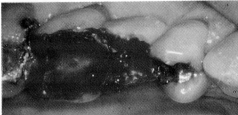

b

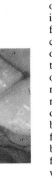

Figure 3.10 (a) Missing 5̲|. It was decided to make a simple cantilever bridge using 6̲| as the abutment. (b) The functional wax recording of opposing cusp movements. The wax is supported on a resin base. (c) A plaster index is made of the wax record. (d) The functional core and the working cast are related on a twin stage occluder. The functional core and the opposing model are mounted on two upper arms. The working model (whether upper or lower) is mounted on the single lower arm of the articulator. (e) The finished bridge is articulated with the functional core. (f) The fitted bridge. Note the supragingival finishing margin of the crown where appearance is not compromised

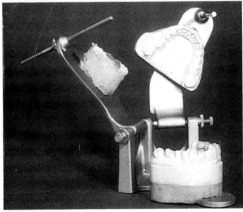

c

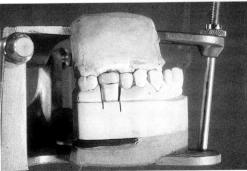

d

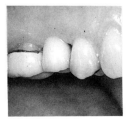

e

f

Table 3.1 Interocclusal records and articulators for specific situations

Restoration type	Occlusal adjustment	Occlusal record	Check	Articulator
Single unit posterior tooth (a) Canine protected occlusion or steep anterior guidance	Only if tooth is initial contact in RCP or there is a NWS contact. Do adjustment at least one visit before tooth preparation. Opposing overerupted teeth may be reduced at the preparation stage	– None or local zinc oxide eugenol paste record (occlusal surface of preparation and opposing cusp tips only) taken with teeth in ICP	Not required if ICP readily identified and stable. Otherwise take a non-wax record. Same teeth that hold Shimstock in mouth should hold Shimstock on casts	Not usually required. Hand held casts suffice if sufficient teeth to occlude casts in stable fashion and it is a posterior tooth that is being crowned
(b) Group function occlusion or shallow anterior guidance	As (a) above	– Local occlusal plaster index made over an FGP wax record intra-orally	Cusp tips of teeth adjacent to the preparation must contact their opposing imprints on the occlusal surface of the trimmed plaster index	Twin stage occluder (Hanau) or semi-adjustable articulator
Single unit anterior tooth	May be indicated if tooth at end of slide RCP→ICP	None or localized record as described above	As above	Not usually required
Single unit posterior tooth copying existing occlusal surface	Not required	– Rigid index of existing tooth or restoration or temporary	Trimmed anatomic index should seat fully before and after wax up and casting	Use a cast relator (Hanau) or hand locate the anatomic index if this can be done reliably
Multiple units/quadrant restoration	As (a) above but may be greater need for occlusal adjustment preoperatively	For quadrant restoration use local record taken in ICP. Use a resin platform (made on a spare cast) relined with ZOE or alternatively use acrylic bonnets. When taking such records for multiple units it is essential that the occlusal vertical dimension be maintained, usually on unprepared or temporized anteriors	Check for tooth contacts in ICP (with Shimstock) in the mouth and confirm on mounted casts after each laboratory phase	Use a suitable semi-adjustable articulator

Chapter 4

Temporary restorations

The preparation of a tooth for an inlay, crown or retainer of a bridge will entail the removal of enamel, the removal of the contact areas with adjacent teeth, the exposure of dentine and the contact with opposing teeth. This will leave the patient with a sensitive and often unsightly tooth, if not protected by a temporary restoration. Furthermore, the loss of contact with adjacent teeth may allow the tooth to move out of its original position and may lead to periodontal or occlusal problems. A temporary cover for the period between tooth preparation and the fitting of the restoration is therefore necessary.

Temporary restorations are not confined to teeth prepared for crowns, but are also an important intermediate stage in the preparation of inlays.

The main functions of temporary restorations are as follows:

1. Protection of the pulp, dentine and any enamel margins exposed during tooth preparation.
2. Stabilization of the tooth to prevent movement.
3. Prevention of gingival overgrowth and the maintenance of gingival health by proper adaptation and contour of the restoration.
4. The maintenance of appearance when used in the anterior region of the mouth.

If pins are to be used for additional retention of the restoration then the pinholes have to be protected by the insertion of a small piece of a paper point so that the temporary cement does not obliterate them.

A number of materials have been used in the past, in conjunction with either polycarbonate or cellulose acetate crown forms, in the construction of temporary crowns. None of these was entirely satisfactory, particularly as far as strength and appearance was concerned.

A chemically-activated composite type of materials, Protemp, which can be used with a variety of shades to alter the final colour, is strong and excellent in appearance when used properly. It can be used for single crowns or multiple units such as bridges with one, two or sometimes even three pontics.

Techniques

Temporary restorations may be made in the laboratory. However, the following techniques are suitable for making them at the chairside.

Figure 4.1 A temporary crown
after removal from the impression
tray. Note the excess material still
attached to the crown, which has
to be carefully removed before
cementation

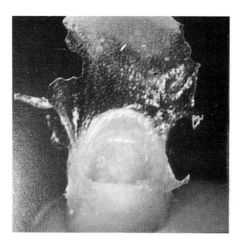

Temporary single units

Before crown preparation, a sectional silicone or alginate impression is
taken of the arch that contains the tooth to be restored. This is then set aside.
If much tooth destruction has taken place prior to preparation, this can be
restored with soft wax to simulate the normal tooth anatomy. After the
impression has been taken, buccal extensions and flanges of the material are
cut away for ease of handling.

After tooth preparation, the temporary crown material is prepared and
syringed into the original impression of the tooth. The tray with the
temporary crown material is then re-inserted into the mouth and held until
almost set. It should be removed when the material is still slightly rubbery.
This usually takes 4 to 5 min. If there is some material left in the syringe this
can be extruded and used to determine the setting time.

On removal of the impression tray from the mouth, the crown, including
some excess, sometimes stays in the impression material but usually remains
on the teeth. It is removed carefully with a probe or small excavator. Care
must be taken to remove all the excess from the mouth, as this is usually in
the form of a thin film and can be missed, which would cause the patient
discomfort (Figure 4.1).

All excess of material is removed from the crown prior to cementation so
that there is no overhang, which might irritate the gingivae. It is imperative
that a temporary restoration does not cause gingival interference or
stagnation areas.

When restoring a single unit there is occasionally a place for the use of an
aluminium crown form. In the posterior region, tooth reduction is
sometimes minimal, and in this situation the aluminium crown form is
stronger and more suitable than composite alternatives. They are easily
adapted to fit the occlusal surfaces and contact areas but care must be taken
to trim the gingival margin so that the metal does not irritate the gingivae.

Temporary post crowns

The construction of a temporary post crown is based on the same principle.
If a matching root canal drill and post system is used, a temporary soft metal

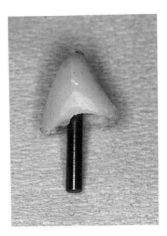

Figure 4.2 A temporary post crown

post is usually included in the system. This is cut to the correct length and fitted to the canal. It should fit accurately.

Alternatively, an impression is taken before the removal of the coronal part of the tooth, or with a stock tooth in place over the root surface of the tooth to be crowned, and set aside. A post made of roughened wire is fitted to the prepared post hole but not cemented. It should project about 2 to 4 mm without interfering with the occlusion on closure of the mouth.

The impression of the tooth to be crowned is now filled with the temporary crown material and inserted over the post in the root canal. On setting it is removed, together with the post firmly embedded in the material. This is trimmed as described above, and the temporary post crown is then ready for cementation (Figure 4.2).

Temporary inlays
For the temporary restoration of inlay preparations a light-cured single component composite resin designed specially for the temporary restoration of inlay cavities can be used. These materials have minimal shrinkage, and remain elastic after curing but are sufficiently hard for adjustment of the occlusion with steel burs. Fermit is one such material. It is easily inserted and adapted to the cavity walls and later easily removed with a probe. However, it has a tendency to discolor after a period and is therefore not very suitable for the anterior region of the mouth.

Temporary bridges
A temporary bridge is constructed in a similar way. The gap to be bridged may be restored by using a stock tooth, which is held in place with soft wax. An alginate or silicone impression is taken over this fragile restoration. The wax and tooth is then removed from the impression prior to the next step. Alternatively, the impression may be made on a study cast that has had a pontic waxed into place.

A temporary restoration can sometimes be used to demonstrate a specific design possibility. This is not always obvious to a patient during discussions about the restorative problem (Figure 4.3).

Figure 4.3 (a) Patient with missing 1|1. There has been drift into the edentulous area. Insufficient space exists for two normal-sized central incisor teeth. (b) Diagnostic wax-up providing three large incisor teeth, which was accepted by the patient. (c) Vacuum-formed stent produced from a diagnostic model for a temporary bridge. (d) Metal ceramic preparations on 2|2. (e) Temporary bridge made of Pro-Temp. (f) Temporary bridge in place. Note the poor connector area appearance, due to the need to overcontour the lateral incisor teeth to close the space. (g) The completed bridge. Gingival-coloured porcelain is used to disguise the proximal areas

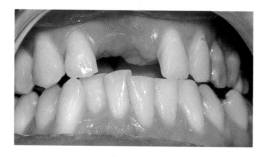

a

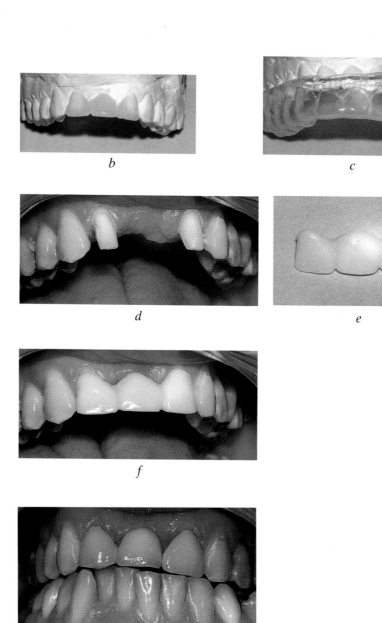

b

c

d

e

f

g

A vacuum-formed shell matrix prepared from a study cast is an excellent alternative method for the construction of a temporary bridge, particularly when a large gap is to be restored. Once again, it is important to remember to remove all the excess material. If there are excessive or large undercuts these must be blocked out before the impression is taken.

If the patient has a denture that is to be replaced by a bridge, this can be used very successfully to fill the pontic area during the impression. In this case, the palatal area of the denture will allow much excess to flow into that area during the re-insertion of the impression tray with the temporary bridge material in place. This must, of course, all be removed together with the excess around the retainers and pontic.

Provisional restorations

Occasionally it is necessary to divide the treatment into stages. Primary restorative treatment may be followed by periodontal treatment before definitive restorations can be prepared and fitted. In such situations, when multiple crowns or extensive bridgework are part of the treatment plan, preliminary crown preparation is often followed by periodontal treatment. The periodontist is helped if the crowns can be removed for better access to the root surfaces of the teeth involved. The provisional crowns will often have to be in place for several weeks until the periodontal treatment is completed. Laboratory-made acrylic crowns are often preferred in such situations because they are stronger and stand up to repeated removal and re-fitting better than those made at the chairside. Such medium- to long-term temporary crowns or bridges are usually called 'provisional restorations'.

When laboratory-made provisional crowns are to be used, the teeth are prepared in the normal way, and before the next step, an alginate impression is taken of the prepared teeth. This is sufficiently accurate for the technician to construct acrylic crowns. An impression of the opposing jaw is also required as well as the selection of the correct shade and a registration of the occlusion.

A major advantage of resin provisional restorations is that they can be modified. The shape can be altered, the shade changed, and the patient has a period during which a decision can be made about the final shape and appearance of the crowns or bridge.

Cementation

Laboratory-made restorations are polished in the laboratory but temporary restorations made at the chairside must be polished at the chairside. Furthermore, a final check of the occlusion and margins must be made because adjustments are simpler before cementation (Figure 4.4).

When either the temporary or provisional crown or bridge is cemented it is best to avoid hard setting cements. There are several proprietary temporary cements on the market and any of these will suffice. Their advantage is that the setting hardness can be varied with the addition of some petroleum jelly. Also, they usually leave the prepared tooth surface very clean.

Figure 4.4 A well-trimmed
temporary bridge prior to
cementation

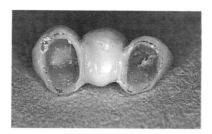

In the case of post crowns, about 1 mm of the temporary post should be
cut off the end to allow a small ball of cotton wool to be inserted into the
post-hole before cementation. This, when later removed with a barbed
broach, will ensure that there is no temporary cement left in the hole, which
might hinder accurate seating of the permanent post.

Chapter 5

Impression materials and techniques

The tooth that has been prepared and finished carefully requires an equally careful impression technique. Reliable materials must be used with some understanding of their limitations. Without this the impression stage can nullify earlier achievements in the preparation.

Visco-elastic (elastomeric) materials are normally used for impressions in inlay, crown and bridge work. They are based on polysulphide, silicone and polyether rubbers; hydrocolloid materials are also available.

Materials

The principal features of the groups of impression materials are described in the following paragraphs and summarized in Table 5.1.

Polysulphides

Polysulphide polymers were the first synthetic rubbers to be used as impression materials and can produce accurate impressions with good stability.

The materials are presented as base and activator pastes of contrasting colours. The activator is lead dioxide. Most brands are available in three viscosities: low, medium and high, which are usually described by the manufacturer as light, regular and heavy bodied. The low and high viscosity materials are intended to be used consecutively. The low viscosity material is injected into the preparation area using a syringe; the high viscosity material, held in a tray, is then placed over the low viscosity material to reinforce its flow into the details of the preparations. As an alternative, medium viscosity material can be used in both the syringe and the tray.

The principal disadvantage of these materials is that they are unpleasant to mix and use. The manipulation time is 3 min and the total setting time is 10 min from the start of mixing, which in some circumstances may be a disadvantage. A particular difficulty has been the formation of subsurface bubbles in the mixed material. These may be a source of local instability as a result of contraction and distortion in a set impression as the gas content of the bubbles disappears. The presence of lead dioxide must focus attention on the toxicity of the impression material but so far there is no evidence to contra-indicate its use. Later polysulphides have copper hydrate or peroxide catalysts and contain less sulphur. They are, therefore, more pleasant for the patient than earlier materials. Their dimensional stability is also considered to be better than those with lead dioxide activators.

Polysulphides are insignificantly affected by normal storage conditions. The shelf life is good and the setting time predictable. Another advantage is their slight hydrophilia so that traces of moisture on the tooth surface will not inhibit the flow of the material. They also have good elasticity and resistance to tearing. These latter qualities are important when taking full-arch impressions, particularly of teeth with long clinical crowns and large interdental spaces, or when segments of the mouth have existing bridge work. Unless a material is sufficiently elastic these conditions may make removal difficult without causing tears in areas of thin section or considerable discomfort to the patient. In the case of polysulphides the danger that teeth will break off the cast model during removal of the impression is avoided.

As with all elastomers, the setting reaction of polysulphides continues over a lengthy period but the most rapid rate of change takes place in the first 10 min. after mixing is complete. The manufacturer chooses an arbitrary time after this most rapid rate of change to recommend as the time for removal of the material from the mouth. However, as with other elastomers, if the material is held in the mouth for longer than this recommended time the permanent deformation following the strains of removal will be less and the dimensional stability of the impression after removal will be greater.

Silicones

These materials are available in viscosities ranging from free-flowing liquids to stiff putties. The majority of them are presented as two-paste systems or as putty and paste. Others, now less commonly in use, consist of a base paste and liquid activator.

The difference stems from the method of polymerization. The earlier version of the silicone material has a liquid activator and a condensation, cross-linking form of polymerization. The more recent type is cured by an increase in length of the polymer chains as well as cross-linkage. This is referred to as addition curing.

Condensation reaction type
Alcohol is a by-product of polymerization and although only formed in small amounts its evaporation causes shrinkage. This may be significant in thin sections of material but is minimal with the heavily filled putties. The total manipulation time is 3 min. and the overall setting time is 6 min.

Addition reaction type
There are no volatile by-products of the reaction to cause dimensional change so the set material is both accurate and stable. It is supplied as a series of two-paste systems with differing viscosities. There are light, regular and heavy bodied varieties as well as a highly viscous putty material. The recommended manipulation time is 3 min. and the overall setting time is 8 min. Because contact with latex gloves can inhibit polymerization of these materials, vinyl gloves should be worn when mixing or handling putties.

Advantages and disadvantages of silicones

The main disadvantage of all silicones is that they are hydrophobic, although some more than others. The prepared surfaces of tooth must, therefore, be clean and completely dry at the time the impression is taken because the material will not flow readily over a moist surface. This is critical at the gingival margin of preparations where it is difficult to eliminate all traces of moisture.

Some silicone materials are stiff when set, particularly the addition-cured type, and this property may lead to the difficulties already discussed when used for full-arch impressions or for several teeth with long clinical crowns. On the other hand, the materials have adequate resistance to tearing and the addition-cured variety has excellent dimensional stability. It is also unaffected by normal conditions of storage and altogether the material is pleasant, clean and easy to use. Copper plating is possible, although the effects on dimensional stability of metal plating have not been fully established.

Polyethers

These materials are marketed as two paste systems, available in various viscosities. The standard manipulation time is 3 min. with a recommended setting time of 6 min. from the start of mixing. The polyether molecule is hydrophilic, which is a source of dimensional changes. It is a stable material if kept completely dry but this is difficult to achieve in dentistry. Dry storage and transit conditions are also critical for limiting dimensional change during transport between surgery and laboratory. It is a stiff material when set but has only a moderate resistance to tearing, which is an unfortunate combination that poses difficulties for full-arch impressions and for teeth with long clinical crowns. The material is, however, clean and easy to handle with a very good shelf life.

Hydrocolloids

The hydrocolloids are of two types: the reversible (agar) type and the irreversible (alginate) type. They both have a high water content and are unstable in the set state because of their tendency to absorb or lose water rapidly. This alteration in water content results in dimensional changes and, therefore, distortion. To minimize this distortion the models must be cast as soon as possible after the impression has been taken. Even if the impression is placed in a humidor to control the change in water content there may still be distortion within 30 min. of the material setting.

Reversible hydrocolloids

Some practitioners favour these materials. This seems to be due mainly to their hydrophilic property, which facilitates the recording of surface detail even in the presence of moisture. The dimensional stability of the set material is clinically acceptable if the model is cast immediately and allowed to set in a humidor. Prior immersion of the impression surface in potassium sulphate solution may be necessary to condition it. The principal difficulty when using this weak material is that it may tear when withdrawn from undercuts. Fine tags of the material in gingival crevices often tear on removal. The system is not convenient for the occasional user because the material has to be prepared first by boiling and then conditioning, a process that may take 30 min to complete. For a regular user, the conditioned material may be kept in a heated storage bath for up to 1 week.

The impression is obtained by an injection of material for cavity detail supplemented by material in a tray. The trays have a water jacket for cooling the material while the impression is held in place.

Irreversible hydrocolloids

The alginates are in common use and there are many proprietary brands available that are accurate enough for use in restorative dentistry. The material sets as a result of a reaction between sodium alginate and calcium sulphate, giving insoluble calcium alginate. The material is weak compared with the synthetic rubbers and in thin section tends to distort or tear on withdrawal of the impression. It is, therefore, contra-indicated as an impression material for tooth preparations. It has a useful role as an impression material for study casts and opposing models for occlusal records.

Choice of impression material

With correct handling and proper preparation of the mouth all the visco-elastic impression materials in current use are capable of providing good impressions. The choice of material is, therefore, largely dependent on personal preference.

Polysulphides have the advantage of being slightly hydrophilic, so can be used in situations where moisture control is difficult. They are easy to manipulate and tear-resistance is excellent but they are less pleasant for the patient than silicones or polyethers.

All silicone materials are hydrophobic, so excellent moisture control is essential for accuracy. They are easy to manipulate, but latex gloves should not be worn when handling them. They are pleasant for the patient and tear-resistance is moderately high.

Polyethers are easy to manipulate and pleasant for the patient but they are stiff when set and can, in some instances, be difficult to remove from the cast.

Reversible hydrocolloids require considerable special equipment and are cumbersome to use. They are, however, hydrophilic and potentially useful in the presence of moisture but the model must be cast immediately.

Irreversible hydrocolloids are not suitable as impression materials for tooth preparations and should only be used for a cast of the opposing jaw and study casts.

Table 5.1 summarizes the principal factors of the visco-elastic impression materials.

Table 5.1 The principal features of visco-elastic impression materials

	Polysulphides	Condensation silicones	Addition silicones	Polyethers	Hydrocolloids	
					Alginate	Agar
Presentation	Regular, heavy and light pastes	Putty, regular and wash pastes	Putty, regular, heavy and light pastes	Regular, heavy and light pastes	Powder	Syringe packs and tray packs
Mixing time	1 min	30 sec	45 sec	45 sec	45 sec	30 min boiling and conditioning
Working time	2 min	1–1.5 min	2 min	2 min	1–1.5 min	
Holding time	7 min	2–3 min	3–5 min	2–3 min	2 min	3–5 min
Total time	10 min	4–5 min	6–8 min	5–6 min	4–5 min	—
Decreased setting time	Raise temperature	Raise temperature. More catalyst	Raise temperature	Raise temperature. More catalyst	Raise temperature	Lower coolant temperature
Dimensional change in setting	0.5–1.5%	0.6%	0.05–0.16%	0.15%	1.5–3.0%	1.0–1.5%
Stiffness after set	Low	Moderate	Moderate	High	Low	Low
Tear resistance	Very high	Moderate–high	Moderate–high	Moderate	Low	Very low
Shelf life	Good	Moderate	Good	Very good	Very good	Very good

Techniques

Gingival margin control

This is critical to the successful use of elastic impression materials and is the most vulnerable part of any technique. Healthy gingival margins must be established beforehand and atraumatic preparation is also an important precondition. Electrosurgery may be useful for recontouring the gingivae and a fine electrode allows the precise removal of very small pieces of tissue. This must be followed by other measures, which will include a gingival pack and the appropriate postoperative supervision. Unless electrosurgery is used with care, however, it is possible to damage the underlying bone, which could lead to pain, necrosis, delayed healing and excessive loss of soft tissue.

Where the gingivae are healthy and the preparation does not extend deeply subgingivally, blowing impression material into the gingival crevice is generally all that is required. However, it may be necessary to pack the crevice to displace the free gingivae. This will open the crevice to the impression material. Ideally 1 mm of tooth surface beyond the margins of the preparation should be accessible for the impression in order to provide a workable model in the laboratory, with the margins clearly defined for the technician.

The teeth and other tissues to be included in the impression must be cleaned and dried. Cleaning the teeth before drying and before gingival retraction helps to remove the saliva film and reduces surface tension. The effect is to promote the flow of the material for a detailed impression. Good saliva control is vital at this stage, using well-placed cotton-wool rolls and effective aspiration.

A variety of cotton cords is available, both plain and impregnated with either adrenaline or an astringent. Modern braided or knitted cords are preferred to the older twisted cords. The latter are prone to separate on packing, in comparison to braided cords, and are more likely to be caught on burs if they are placed before preparation margins are finished. The smallest cord that allows displacement of the gum 0.5 mm apical to the preparation margin should be chosen. Stiffer cords provide greater horizontal tissue displacement but are more prone to rebound on packing and have less capacity to absorb retraction chemicals. Adrenaline 0.1% impregnated cord affords good haemostasis, tissue displacement and minimal gingival irritation/recession. However, adrenaline may cause adverse systemic effects and this type of cord should not be used on susceptible patients or when the tissue has been lacerated. Astringent solutions, such as aluminium sulphate, aluminium chloride, ferric sulphate or zinc chloride, are also useful for obtaining haemostasis and/or tissue displacement.

It is important that cord of the appropriate thickness is chosen. It is packed into the gingival crevice using a flat plastic instrument. The cord is held in a light loop around the tooth and tucked carefully but firmly between tooth and free gingivae, starting where the cord can be retained (e.g. interdentally) and preferably where the margin is supragingival. Alternatively, two plastic instruments may be used, one to hold the cord down and the other to tuck it into the crevice (Figure 5.1).

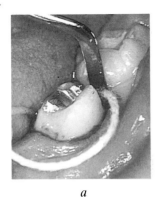
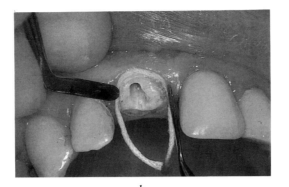

a   *b*

Figure 5.1 (a) Retraction cord is tucked carefully between tooth and gingivae. (b) Two plastic instruments may be helpful in retaining the cord during packing

A careful check should be made that all the foregoing procedures have been completed successfully. If not, it is important not to proceed, but to postpone the impression until gingival health has been improved or satisfactory moisture control gained, or both. During the intervening period a well-fitting temporary restoration should be placed.

Impression trays

For polysulphides and many silicones, a laboratory-made special tray is required. This is normally constructed on a study cast. The tray may be made from a variety of materials but a self-curing acrylic resin is probably the strongest. It should be adapted to allow about 2 to 3 mm of impression material between the teeth and the tray. The tray must be sufficiently rigid to avoid distortion in use. A small projection is required on each side together with a firmly attached handle. These will assist rapid removal of the tray with the completed impression. It is also advisable to include three occlusal stops distributed over unprepared teeth in the arch to maintain the spacing.

Spacing is important to provide an adequate bulk of flexible material. This is particularly so in the neighbourhood of undercuts, to ensure recovery from the strains developed during removal of the impression. It will also minimize the chance of tears. Excessive bulk may lead to polymerization shrinkage.

A stock tray is used for polyether materials. Stock trays are also used for putty and paste techniques, because the putty provides the necessary adaptation to the teeth, and for alginate impressions.

If disposable stock trays are used they should be made of polycarbonate, which is more rigid than some other plastics used for the manufacture of impression trays.

Impression techniques

Some thought should be given to the information that it is expected to record in an impression. The following list may help:

1. Details of the prepared tooth tissue including, if possible, at least 1 mm of normal tissue beyond the margins.

2. The surfaces of adjacent teeth that will be in contact with the planned restorations.
3. The occlusal surfaces of teeth in the arch.
4. The form and shape of the arch.
5. Soft-tissue surfaces in the area of a bridge pontic.

Filling a tray with impression material and placing it in the mouth will not record all the information accurately. None of the elastic impression materials will displace the gingivae to reach a subgingival margin. Also, air may be trapped under such an impression, particularly within an intracoronal section of a preparation.

To overcome these difficulties a syringe is used to inject a mix into all the details of a preparation, which is then followed by the main mass held in a tray. This injection method can be used with any of the elastic materials.

Injection technique

While the mouth is being prepared, the chosen impression material should have been dispensed on a mixing pad by an assistant.

The fitting surface of the tray should be coated with a thin layer of appropriate adhesive solution. The adhesive should be carried over the periphery of the tray for about 2 mm. This ensures that the impression material is retained firmly in the tray upon removal. The adhesive should be allowed to dry for sufficient time before the material is loaded into the tray. All materials should be mixed according to the manufacturer's directions. For silicone materials, two mixes are prepared: the syringe mix is undertaken by the operator and begun about 30 sec before the tray mix, which is prepared by an assistant. The operator loads the first mix into the syringe as quickly as possible and removes the gingival packs and cotton-wool rolls. The material must be injected into all parts of the cavity with the syringe nozzle in the deepest part, filling from its depth to the surface. The nozzle is always kept within the bulk of the material, and corners where air is likely to be trapped are given special attention (Figure 5.2). It may help to use compressed air to distribute the elastic material around a preparation after an initial application. Meanwhile, the assistant

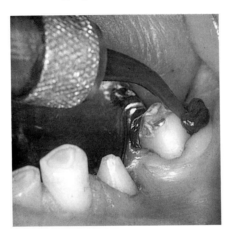

Figure 5.2 Injection material being injected around the prepared tooth. Note the tapered preparation, which is not ideal

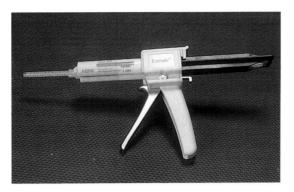

Figure 5.3 Automixing syringe

loads the second mix in the tray, which is then seated in position, after being coated with a thin layer of wash material, and held firmly until the material is set.

Uniformity in colour is an indication that the material has been fully mixed. An alternative to mixing by hand is the use of an automixer (Figure 5.3). These devices operate by pushing the catalyst and the base through a special tip containing vanes that mix the material. This is easier than mixing by hand and the material contains less voids. Automixers are used predominantly with addition-cured silicone materials.

Putty and paste technique

When it is certain that the margins of the preparation will be easy to record, the putty and wash are used in a single stage. After the tray has been loaded, it is helpful to mould a trough in the putty, the width of the prepared and adjacent teeth, into which some of the syringe material is placed. This is in addition to syringing some around the prepared teeth.

In more complex situations a two-stage technique is used. In this case the tray should be loaded and seated as soon as the putty is mixed and allowed to set in the mouth for 5 min. After removal from the mouth the impression is washed and dried thoroughly to allow the perfecting paste to bond to its surface. The paste is loaded into the putty tray and some paste may also be syringed into the prepared teeth. The tray is seated with firm pressure, but it is essential that this pressure is released after a few seconds to allow elastic recovery of the putty before the paste begins to set. There may be distortion if this is not done. The material should then be left in the mouth until fully set.

Pins and post-holes

Adequate support is necessary for elastic impressions of any small-bore holes and may be provided by a piece of wire or a matching plastic impression pin. These should be coated with adhesive on the part that projects from the preparation.

Removal and assessment

Impressions using visco-elastic material are best removed from the mouth by a 'snap' action. This is because the rate at which strains are applied to these

Figure 5.4 Rubber base impression, showing complete record of preparations and crevicular areas

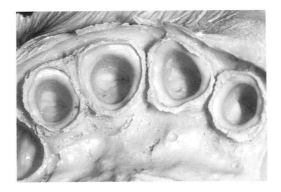

materials affects their elastic recovery. A high rate of applied strains results in good recovery so that snap removal allows elastic recovery to take place rapidly afterwards. The completed impression must be washed clean and dried. It is then scrutinized to ensure that all the details required are recorded (Figure 5.4). It is not always possible to obtain an impression that is free from minor defects in all areas. Naturally, no defect can be accepted in the region of the margins of the preparation but one or two small blow holes well away from the margins may be acceptable.

If the impression is not satisfactory it should be re-taken completely because attempts at improving individual areas by the addition of further material rarely succeed.

Finally, the mouth is re-examined and any torn pieces of material are removed from gingival crevices or interdental spaces.

Locating the die

In addition to an impression of the prepared teeth it is necessary to be able to place this accurately in relation to adjacent and opposing teeth on models. It is important, however, that an adequate number of teeth are included in the impression. The most satisfactory way of ensuring this and subsequent accuracy in the laboratory is by the use of impressions of the whole prepared arch, which can be occluded with a cast made of the opposing arch.

Registration of the occlusion gives the relationship of the prepared teeth to the opposing arch. Descriptions of methods of recording these relationships are given in Chapter 3.

Making crowns fit existing removable partial dentures

It is often necessary to make (or remake) a crown for a tooth serving as a removable partial denture abutment. If the existing removable partial denture is to continue to serve satisfactorily then it is necessary to make the new crown to fit the removable appliance accurately in areas of rest seats, retentive clasp arms, bracing arms or guide planes.

This may be accomplished by constructing a crown in pattern resin (Duralay: Reliance Dent. Mfg. Co., Worth Ill., USA) on the working model. On the first visit an alginate impression is taken of the prepared tooth with the partial denture *in situ*, together with a master silicone impression for model and die construction. With the aid of the cast from the alginate impression, a pattern is made in resin on a duplicate of the master die. At the second visit this is tried in and selective adjustment is made, either removing areas of excess contour or building up areas deficient in contour (with direct pattern wax or with more resin using the brush/bead technique) before returning the pattern to the laboratory for casting and finishing. The final crown is then fitted on the third visit.

Materials for direct impressions

Casting wax. The type of wax chosen by the practitioner will be decided partly by individual preference and this, to a large extent, is formed by experience. However, one important feature is the need to use a high melting point wax for direct patterns. Otherwise the pattern will remain soft at mouth temperature and be difficult to carve to a fine margin. It will also distort readily.

Acrylic resin. It may often be preferable to use an acrylic resin material for a direct pattern. For example, when additional strength of the pattern is required before removal from the mouth. Special materials (Duralay: Reliance Dent. Mfg. Co., Worth Ill., USA) have been manufactured for taking impressions. When heated in investment these burn out completely, leaving no residue.

Direct technique

Although used rarely it should be remembered that it is possible to produce a pattern 'directly' in the mouth. With this technique there are few intermediate steps and the laboratory procedures are limited so there is little chance of distortion of the pattern. Practice is, however, necessary to develop skill in carving in the mouth and care is required in the subsequent handling of the pattern. The direct technique may be suitable for simple inlay cavities where access is good, but it is most commonly used for direct patterns for posts and cores in crown work.

Some finishing of the casting is required in the mouth because there is no die and therefore more time is spent at the chairside than for the indirect technique. A direct pattern is not easy to manipulate in thin section, which makes it unsuitable for cuspal coverage or where other surfaces need a thin layer of the pattern.

Decontamination and storage of impressions

There is little evidence of transmission of infection by means of impressions from the mouth, but this does not absolve the clinician from ensuring that proper steps are taken to avoid cross-infection.

Recommendations on this topic change periodically because no universally applicable procedure has yet been devised and unfortunately some disinfectants distort impression materials or degrade surface detail.

The most generally accepted advice is that silicone, polysulphide and direct impressions should be immersed in 1% sodium hypochlorite solution for 30 min but hydrocolloids for not more than 1 min. Glutaraldehyde 2% solution is suggested for polyether.

Most impressions may be cast as soon as convenient after disinfection; with hydrocolloids immediate casting is essential to prevent distortion. All other materials should be dried before storage if they cannot be cast straight away.

Chapter 6

Cementation

The choice of cementing medium can significantly affect the success of inlays, crowns and bridges. A variety of materials is available and therefore the main properties of the various categories of cements are summarized in Table 6.1. Resin retained bridges, veneers and tooth-coloured inlays all have specific techniques for their cementation; these are discussed in the relevant chapters. However, basic principles will be covered here.

Try-in

Upon return from the laboratory a restoration should be checked to ensure the correct design requested has been followed, that the fit on the master die is good and that the contours appear to be correct. The provisional restoration is removed and the preparation carefully checked to ensure complete removal of any temporary cement. A local anaesthetic may be required. The preparation is then dried and isolated.

The restoration is carefully seated onto the preparation, care being taken not to push too hard. If it fails to seat fully, the contact points should initially be checked with dental floss as a tight contact is the most common cause of this problem. The floss should just catch lightly as it is passed through the contact.

Heavier contacts are gently eased until correct. Graphite or Occlude (Pascal, USA) placed on the area will rub off with a tight contact, which can then easily be identified. If the restoration still fails to seat, the fit surface of the casting should be examined for imperfections. A pressure indicating film, such as a silicone fit checker, can be placed on the fit surface and will rub off in an area of tight contact, which can then be relieved. Once the restoration has been seated it can be evaluated for fit, contour and appearance.

Fit

A sharp probe is run around the margins to check for marginal discrepancies. A fit of between 50 to 75 μm is acceptable and at this level of gap an exploratory sharp probe will detect the margin, whereas a greater marginal gap will allow a probe to enter and is therefore unacceptable. A few exceptions exist. For example, if the margin is a thin veneer of gold then it may be possible to burnish down the gold under pressure to close the marginal gap.

Table 6.1 Comparison of cements for luting

Cement	Setting time	Film thickness	Pulpal irritation	Compressive strength	Tensile strength	Solubility
Zinc phosphate	Short	Thin	Moderate	Very high	High	Very low
Fortified zinc oxide/eugenol (polymer reinforced)	Medium	Moderately thin	Very mild	Fairly high	Fairly high	Very low
EBA	Long	Thin	Mild	High	Fairly high	Very low
Zinc polycarboxylate	Short	Thin	Mild	High	Very high	Low
Resin	Variable	Variable	Severe*	High	High	Very low
Glass ionomer	Short	Thin	Mild	High	Very high	Very low

Note. Figures given by different authors for actual values of setting time, film thickness, strength and solubility vary considerably so trends are given instead. In all cases it should be remembered that these are appropriate to mixes used for luting and that values for thicker mixes will be considerably different.
* If used without bonding agent.

In some cases, the fit of a porcelain jacket crown in the mid-palatal area is poor due to the technical process of manufacture. As this area is generally accessible for cleaning and inspection this is generally acceptable. It should be remembered that an open margin means a wide exposure of the cement lute and this in turn may lead to premature failure of the lute and crown, an increased risk of caries at the margin and a possible increase in the accumulation of plaque and therefore periodontal disease. Overbuilt margins should also be detected and adjusted before fitting. An underbuilt or negative margin may be accepted as long as no marginal gap exists and the area is accessible for cleaning.

Finally the fit should be evaluated with regard to tightness and stability of the restoration. A loose fit will require a thick cement lute and lead to an increased chance of failure.

Contour

The contacts should be light as described. Buccal and lingual contours must not be overbuilt and should resemble those of adjacent teeth. The embrasure space is shaped to allow easy access for cleaning, particularly to interdental devices. Occlusal contacts are then checked as described in Chapter 3.

The occlusion is adjusted until light contacts are present in intercuspal relationship. The lateral and protrusive movements are checked and made smooth with no premature contacts and the movement from retruded contact to intercuspal position should not be altered.

Appearance

This is evaluated jointly with the patient. With complex or extensive cases it is wise to have a preliminary try-in of the porcelain at a biscuit bake stage. Any alterations to colour and contour can then be made before glazing. The porcelain shade can be altered by the use of stains in the glaze. It is not possible to lighten a shade, but darkening, yellowing, greying and the provision of characterization, such as incisal translucency, mottling and cracks, can all be incorporated although they are best included in the original prescription.

The labial contour can also significantly affect the appearance and care should be taken with the incisal tip of anterior teeth to get the correct level. Mesial and distal corners should also be correctly shaped.

Before final cementation the patient should be quite happy with the feel, appearance and occlusion of a restoration. Any adjusted areas are repolished but if major alterations to the contour have been necessary, the restoration will need to be returned to the laboratory for re-glazing.

A large mirror and plenty of time to ensure the patient does not feel hurried, are essential for the final agreement on shade and contour before cementation.

Trial cementation

With extensive restorations it is sometimes wise to cement the work provisionally to ensure that all is correct before final and irrevocable cementation. As well-fitting restorations may be difficult to remove, even with very weak cement underneath, this is best undertaken only when deemed essential. A specific trial cement such as modified Temp-bond (Kerr UK Ltd., Peterborough) or Opotow trial cement (Teledyne Getz, Illinois, USA) should be used.

Choice of cement

As will be seen from the footnote to Table 6.1, varying results have been given for the different cements so it is only possible to indicate trends. Even so, it should be remembered that these are based on laboratory tests, which relate to specimens of greater thickness than those used for cementation of restorations. However carefully these tests are undertaken, they cannot simulate performance in the mouth.

On the basis of clinical experience the authors continue to use zinc phosphate for cementing the majority of their restorations, although glass ionomer cements are equally acceptable clinically.

Zinc oxide/eugenol cements, whether reinforced by polymers or EBA, are not commonly used for permanent cementation but may be useful for teeth that are very sensitive, provided the preparations have adequate retention. Polycarboxylate cements, in spite of their good results in laboratory tests, have proved to be disappointing in clinical use and are not generally recommended.

Zinc phosphate cements have a long proven record for clinical success and continue to be the cements by which others are judged. They have acceptable strength, working time, biological properties, and are very easy to handle. Glass ionomer cements have high strength with good retentive properties and low final solubility. The biological properties are superior to those of zinc phosphate. On the negative side, they are harder to mix, have a short working time and should be kept dry during the setting period to prevent a weakened surface layer.

Cementation technique

Whichever cementing medium is chosen, it is essential that it is mixed correctly and that the preparations are dry and free from saliva and debris at the time of cementation.

The restoration is coated with a thin layer of cement, which has been mixed to a creamy 'stringing' consistency. Speed is essential as the restoration must be fully seated before the cement starts to set so that as thin a layer of cement as possible is obtained.

With a well-fitting restoration, a considerable amount of hydrostatic pressure can build up within the cement during seating. If the seating pressure is released before the cement has hardened there can be a rebound of the restoration, resulting in a thicker cement lute. Simply getting the patient to apply pressure to the restoration through closing is not acceptable and the operator should use firm and continued finger pressure on the restoration until satisfied that the cement is hard. Various mechanical devices have been proposed to assist with seating, such as an automatic mallet, but their complexity is not normally required.

Cement release channels are sometimes provided within manufactured parallel-sided posts to allow for excess cement to be easily extruded and reduce the pressure build-up within the tooth.

Excess cement is chipped away from the margins only when it has set fully. Premature removal of excess can result in deficient cement at margins. Floss is used to remove excess proximal cement. The margins of a setting glass ionomer cement should be protected from moisture using unfilled resin.

Finally, the occlusion should be rechecked and the patient instructed in cleaning techniques relative to the new restoration.

Resin-retained restorations

These are dealt with specifically in the relative chapters. However, there are general principles to be followed, essential to the success for the whole of this generation of restorations.

1. Moisture control is paramount and is only guaranteed when a rubber dam is used.
2. Enamel to be used for etch bonding must be clean and plaque-free before etching and should have the characteristic 'frosted' appearance after etching, washing and drying. Poor quality enamel or resistant enamel that has not frosted must be re-treated.
3. Wherever possible, enamel must be used for bonding rather than dentine, particularly at the margins of restorations. The mechanical bond produced to etched enamel is many times stronger and longer lasting than any chemical bond that may be obtained to dentine.
4. It is important to check for excess cement, which is often difficult to see as it may be tooth coloured, and to ensure that the proximal contacts adjacent to the restoration are free from excess.
5. These 'adhesive' techniques are recent and undergoing continuous evolution. It is essential to keep abreast of new techniques and manufacturer's recommendations for new materials carefully.

Chapter 7

Restoration of anterior teeth

The porcelain jacket crown

A porcelain jacket crown consists of a layer of porcelain which covers the whole of the clinical crown of the tooth. In order to accommodate this layer, some of the enamel and dentine of the tooth has to be removed. This type of crown is usually restricted to the anterior region of the mouth.

Indications and contra-indications

The improvement of the patient's appearance is by far the most common indication for the use of porcelain jacket crowns for the restoration of anterior teeth. Loss of part or the whole of the tip of a tooth through trauma is a common reason for the use of jacket crowns. Slight changes in the shape and size of anterior teeth can be achieved by the use of porcelain jacket crowns. Teeth that have suffered from hypoplasia of the enamel can have their appearance totally changed by the use of porcelain jacket crowns.

Although composite restorations and veneers may be acceptable alternatives to jacket crowns in certain situations, the porcelain jacket has been in use for many decades. It is still an aesthetically pleasing and durable restoration, and is the treatment of choice in many instances.

All types of crown have some contra-indications, and the porcelain jacket crown is no exception. It is not suitable for very young patients because of the amount of tooth tissue that has to be removed to accommodate the porcelain. Furthermore, the brittleness of the material makes it unsuitable for those engaged in contact sports.

Specific considerations

One of the specific considerations is the need to accommodate 1 to 2 mm of porcelain without endangering the pulp and without altering the shape of the crown. The patient's lip line is an important factor because it influences the decision about the exact placement of the labial crown margin. Those patients who can not retract their upper lip sufficiently to expose their gingival margins under conditions such as normal speech or smiling, could well do without subgingival margin placement.

Furthermore, the choice of a veneer restoration as an alternative must be considered seriously before embarking on the extensive preparation of the tooth for a jacket crown.

Some of the problems with crown preparation are associated with lack of patient cooperation. Time should be taken beforehand to discuss the procedure with the patient. This discussion should include the time necessary and the fact that a temporary crown of reasonable appearance and function will be placed on the tooth while the permanent crown is being made.

If marginal gingivitis is present, the patient should be warned that the procedure will have to be delayed until this is under control. Soft tissue control for anterior crown impressions, where the labial margin is placed within the gingival crevice, is possibly the most difficult part of the whole procedure. There is always a possibility of a faulty impression if the gum at the margin of the preparation bleeds easily. The importance of good gingival health before crown preparation has been stressed in Chapter 2.

The material

Dental porcelains are basically glass that consists of a mixture of oxides dominated by silicon oxide. This combination of oxides is found in the mineral feldspar, hence feldspathic porcelains, but the mixture of oxides can also be combined synthetically. This permits variation of the oxide mix, which can alter the fusing temperature, viscosity and vitrification of the glass. The manufacturer plans the correct mix of oxides, which are then made into a 'frit' by quenching a superheated glass mix rapidly in cold water.

It is therefore possible to make a range of porcelain with different fusing temperatures. A high temperature fusing porcelain (1250–1350°C) can be a combination of feldspar (85%) and quartz (15%). A low temperature fusing (800–1050°C) and medium temperature fusing (1050–1070°C) porcelains also exist.

Improved translucency is obtained by diminishing the quantity of entrapped air bubbles. This is achieved by fusing powders of small particle size at reduced pressure, generally referred to as vacuum firing.

The strength of porcelain may be improved by including aluminium oxide (alumina) in the oxide mixture. This has the ability to raise the critical tensile strength from 5000 psi to 20 000 psi in high alumina porcelains.

Particle size, shape and proportion of alumina will all affect the ultimate strength of the fused porcelain. Vacuum firing and a strict firing schedule are essential to the strength of aluminous porcelains. High-strength material contains up to 50% alumina of fine grain size. Unfortunately, this material is opaque and its use is therefore limited to forming the core of the crown. Even as a core it may reflect too much light at the interface with the more superficial porcelain so more glass is added to prevent this. The outer layers of a high-alumina crown, representing enamel and dentine, will therefore usually contain more glass to give the translucency required.

One of the dynamic features of porcelain fracture is the rapid propagation of micro-defects into major fracture lines. In feldspathic porcelains, this crack propagation can be reduced by preserving the integrity of the glaze. A high alumina core will help to prevent the propagation of cracks from the internal surface of the crown.

Correct design of the preparation will help to avoid stress concentration by ensuring that there are no sharp angles and no wedge-shaped incursions into the crown shape. Ideally, the crown should have an even thickness throughout. Where this is not possible, the change in thickness should be curved and gradual. Resistance to stress from opposing teeth should be provided by the preparation so that there are no high-tensile stresses but only compressive stresses.

Alternative porcelains have been used with varying degrees of success. For example:

1. Cast glass ceramic systems are methods of producing crowns by casting the material in a very similar way to that used for gold crowns. Marginal adaptation of the castings compares favourably to that of metal crowns.
2. The high-ceram technique, which is based on the refractory die system, has produced a more successful, exceedingly strong all porcelain crown. The system used now is a modification of the original idea and produces a crown with good marginal adaptation and excellent physical properties.

The preparation

Principles

The object of the jacket crown preparation on anterior teeth is to provide sufficient thickness of porcelain for strength and appearance without causing damage to the pulp. At the same time sufficient retention must be provided by the form of the opposing axial walls. This is not easy because the natural taper of anterior teeth can lead to a very conical preparation. Therefore it is essential to regard the cervical third of the tooth as a collar in which the axial walls have a combined taper of about 5°. Sufficient tooth must be removed palatally to allow a minimum thickness of 1 mm of porcelain between the preparation and the opposing teeth in all functional movements. Reduction of the labial face should be sufficient to allow the porcelain to achieve the translucency essential for a natural appearance. Again, this should not be less than 1 mm.

The preparation of the incisal edge will determine the length of the preparation and therefore the essential resistance form. A short preparation will reduce retention, as shown in Figure 7.1, and provide insufficient

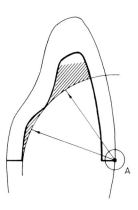

Figure 7.1 If the shaded areas are removed during preparation, retention will be lost between the labial and palatal surfaces and the crown will tend to rotate about point A

Figure 7.2 Insufficient height of the preparation may lead to fractures

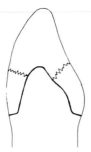

support for the porcelain at the incisal edge. This might cause tensile stresses to develop in the crown, which may lead to its fracture (Figure 7.2). About 2 mm of the incisal edge should be removed.

Sharp junctions between the labial and palatal faces at the incisal edge of the preparation will lead to adverse stress concentrations and propagation of fracture lines in the porcelain.

Insufficient removal of tooth tissue from the labial surface may encourage the technician to overbuild the crown in order to gain sufficient thickness of porcelain for translucency. Failure to reproduce the natural contour of the tooth will make it difficult to prevent gingival inflammation. This is a problem when the gingival margin of the crown is too close to the periodontal attachment. When it is necessary to disguise the gingival margin of a crown, this should be placed no further than half the depth of the gingival crevice. Furthermore, failure to reproduce the natural contour of the tooth will have an adverse effect on the appearance.

It is important to avoid all sharp angles, both internally and externally, as well as those at the incisal edge. Therefore, the junction between the aproximal and other surfaces should be rounded to avoid the generation of internal stresses within the porcelain.

The cavo-surface angle at the gingival margin is 90° to allow sufficient thickness of porcelain at this line for appearance and to avoid weak margins of the crown.

Points for consideration

It is all too easy to remove an excess of tissue quickly and irrevocably at the first stage of preparation, so that time spent in forethought is essential. Some of the problems are as follows:

1. Failure to appreciate that the cutting angle of a tapered diamond point must be controlled in two planes, that is anteroposterior and mesiodistal, which can lead to an exaggerated taper that follows the angle of the incisal two-third. Retention depends on near parallelism in the gingival third of the preparation forming a collar in this area of the tooth.
2. If the palatal surface is prepared before the labial surface, too much tissue may be removed so that the labial face of the preparation has to be kept forward, leaving insufficient space for the porcelain.
3. Too much incisal reduction of the tooth will remove support needed as resistance form for the porcelain.

4. Cutting into the cingulum area from the labial approach will cause an unequal width of shoulder and loss of some retention form.
5. Placing the gingival margin of the preparation too deeply into the gingival crevice labially may result in permanent gingivitis, even with good oral hygiene.
6. Placing the palato-gingival margin too high on the palatal surface may result in loss of valuable retention form.

The stages of tooth preparation

1. *Labial cervical collar* (Figure 7.3)

Use a coarse tapered point to establish the gingival margin of the preparation just coronal to the gingival crest. A shoulder is produced that is at least 1 mm wide. A hand-held number 2 fissure bur may be used as a width gauge for this critical stage. It is 1 mm in diameter. The angle of the cut should be in the long axis of the tooth and will form part of the axial retention collar in the gingival third of the clinical crown.

The remainder of the preparation follows closely on the preparation at the gingival margin and will terminate at the approximal contact areas. Some operators may like to cut orientation grooves to a depth of 1 mm to ensure a correct amount of labial tooth reduction during stage 4.

2. *Palatal cervical collar* (Figure 7.4)

The same procedure is now followed on the palatal surface to produce an angle of 5° to the prepared labial surface.

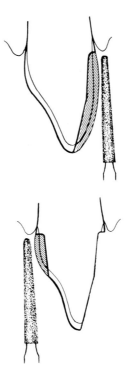

Figure 7.3 Preparation of the labial surface showing two distinct angles. Stage 1 involves the preparation of a cervical collar whilst that of the remaining labial surface is carried out as stage 4

Figure 7.4 Preparation of the palatal surface to form part of the cervical collar at stage 2

Figure 7.5 Preparation of the approximal surface at stage 3

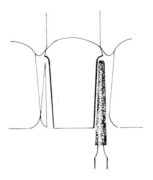

3. *Approximal surfaces* (Figure 7.5)
Place the tip of the tapered diamond point level with the gingival crest and keep the body of the point within tooth tissue. The labial and the palatal surfaces are joined. The angle of the cut should not exceed 5° to the long axis of the tooth and should produce an even depth of shoulder following the natural curves of the tooth. It is important not to allow the diamond point to drift into the cingulum area and thereby remove too much tooth (Figure 7.6). As the point moves from the labial to the palatal surface it should follow the rise and fall of the contour formed by the interdental papilla. However, with a long interdental papilla there will be a wedge-shaped incursion into the porcelain crown periphery, which will cause stress concentration. Modifying the approximal gingival margin to produce a more gentle curve will lessen the chance of adverse stress concentration. A common fault at this stage is to incline the prepared axial surfaces more than the acceptable 5° taper towards the midline, thereby losing retention and endangering the pulpal horns. Retaining the incisal edge throughout these early stages will assist the inexperienced operator to avoid some of these errors.

4. *Remainder of labial surface* (Figure 7.3)
As retention is assured by the preparation of the cervical collar on the labial surface it is only necessary to remove enough tooth from the incisal two-thirds to accommodate an adequate thickness of porcelain. If orientation grooves were cut during stage 1, then it is only necessary to remove sufficient tooth substance to the base of the depth of the orientation groove.

5. *The remainder of the palatal and incisal surfaces*
The cervical collar has already been prepared for retention so the object of this stage is to remove sufficient tooth from the incisal two-thirds of the palatal surface to allow a minimum of 1 mm clearance between the prepared tooth and the opposing teeth in maximum intercuspation and all functional

Figure 7.6 The danger of excessive tooth removal during stage 3 is shown at (A). The correct angulation of the approximal cut is shown at (B)

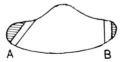

A   B

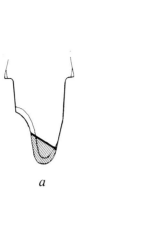 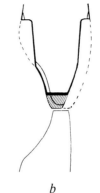

a   b

Figure 7.7 Shortening the length of the tooth for (a) normal incisor relationship and (b) edge to edge incisor relationship

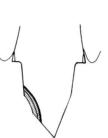

Figure 7.8 The curved palatal reduction is achieved with a large round diamond

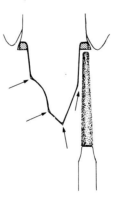

Figure 7.9 The margin is placed within the gingival crevice and the remaining sharp angles are rounded with a fine grade diamond point

movements of the mandible. As part of the same stage incisal clearance can also be established. Here approximately 2 mm of clearance is necessary to leave sufficient support for the crown and yet, at the same time, allow translucency at the incisal edge of the crown (Figure 7.7).

This tooth removal may be carried out with a large round diamond (Figure 7.8). Clearance should be tested with wax wafers if there is any doubt.

6. *Finishing and establishing the final gingival margin* (Figure 7.9)
At this stage the final level of the labial gingival margin is established within the gingival crevice for a satisfactory appearance. All sharp angles left from previous stages are rounded to finish the preparation (Figures 7.10 and

Figure 7.10 Cross-section of an upper incisor showing the approximal reduction and the start of the shoulder on the labial and palatal aspects. The arrows indicate the four points at which discing may be necessary at the angle shown by the dotted lines

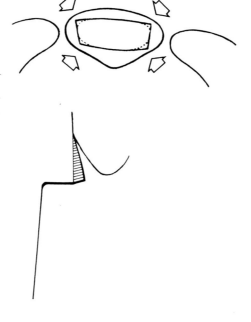

Figure 7.11 Removal of any unsupported enamel at the gingival margin

7.11). Although a plain cut tungsten-carbide bur can be used, it is very easy to dig grooves with this instrument unless it is used with delicate care. The finest grade of diamond points with rounded ends are easier to use and just as efficient. Unsupported enamel at the cervical margin is removed with a hand trimmer (Figure 7.11).

Impressions and occlusal registration

Elastic impression materials are used for taking impressions of the prepared teeth. Control of the gingival crevice is also required to avoid distortion of the margin due to overhanging gingiva, blood or moisture.

If the decision is made to work with partial rather than full arch impression trays, then it is essential that the partial impression is accompanied by functional as well as static occlusal records. Great care is required by the technician when laying down platinum foil on a 'stone' model as all the sharp margins reproduced in the model are extremely vulnerable to wear. The techniques of gingival control and impression taking are described in earlier chapters.

The opposing teeth
A full alginate impression of the opposing dentition will be necessary for the majority of patients. A cast of all teeth of the opposing jaw will more readily allow occlusal clearance to be checked but will not supply information about the functional movements. Two hand-held casts will in many cases give the technician sufficient indication of the occlusion, and will enable the recording of contacts in all movements. This will ensure that the crown does not interfere in protrusive and lateral excursions.

Appearance

An anterior crown of unsatisfactory appearance, however good its fit, will be considered a failure and yet this feature is probably the most difficult on which to offer clear advice. A systematic approach to the problems of colour, shape and surface characteristics is essential, but it is still vulnerable to inaccurate interpretation and poor artistic execution by the technician.

Colour

The ability to select an accurate colour and shade match varies considerably between individuals and the following advice will only compensate partially for the lack of flair.

Because porcelains are metameric, that is they give different colour appearances with different light radiations, advice is usually given that a colour should be judged in daylight. This is the commonest light source for viewing the finished crown and logically the best light for colour selection. However, the limited hours of daylight in the northern hemisphere, especially during winter, together with its varying colour temperature make this advice impractical for many dentists. One constant light source is offered by the quartz-iodine operating light provided this is kept free of dust. Alternatively, a separate light with constant colour temperature (7000 Kelvin) can be used. The light should fall evenly, without lip-shadow, upon the teeth which are dried to avoid unwanted highlights. Colour distractions such as lipstick should be removed or obscured.

The colour should be chosen at the initial examination and reviewed before the preparation. It is a mistake to select a colour following the preparation when the eyes are fatigued.

The first decision is to determine into which colour group the main body of the tooth belongs, that is white, yellow, brown or grey. From the selected colour group the correct light or dark shade is chosen. The eye rapidly attempts to balance out minor differences of shade so that this stage should not be prolonged. To help the eye it is better to choose a shade that is obviously too light and then follow with one that is obviously too dark. From these two it is then easier to move to more subtle distinctions. Unfortunately, many manufactured shade guides do not provide sufficient examples in each colour group to allow this technique. Furthermore, the guide samples are solid whereas the finished crown is thin in section and may therefore appear lighter than the selected guide. Because this stage is so important to successful crown construction it may be worth the cost of a specially constructed shade guide.

If the neck and tip colours on the shade guide are acceptable it is most helpful to use these because complex modifying instructions can be interpreted correctly only with a long-standing rapport between dentist and technician. When additional instructions are necessary they should be unambiguous such as 'no translucency required in the tip' or 'no difference of neck colour required'.

Remarkable effects can be achieved with the addition of low-fusing glass stains added after the main bake, but such additions should not be attempted unless the technician can see the patient. They are certainly not intended to correct faulty colour selection.

Shape

In many cases it will be possible to judge the overall crown shape from the adjacent standing teeth on the study cast. However, incorrect preparation may encourage overcontouring in the laboratory in an attempt to gain adequate thickness of porcelain. It is a common fault to exaggerate the convexity of the crown at the gingival margin even with adequate shoulder width. This may contribute to a persistent marginal gingivitis even when the oral hygiene is otherwise adequate.

Other areas of importance are the correct approximal contour and the placement of the contact areas so that healthy interdental papillae may be accommodated and maintained in health. Incisal edges and approximal corners must match the adjacent teeth because any mismatch can be seen immediately. Neglect of these important considerations is why so many porcelain crowns appear clumsy and thick compared to their natural neighbours.

Surface characteristics

Highlights can be seen easily on a wet tooth and should correspond to the contours seen on the study cast. Heightening these contours by covering the plaster with colloidal graphite and wiping off is helpful.

A common fault is to place the greatest convexity of the labial face in the midline of the crown rather than towards the approximal surfaces.

It can be satisfying to create the correct shape and surface characteristics in the mouth with the crown at the biscuit bake stage and the foil still in place. This is done with diamonds and white abrasive points on a wet and washed surface, but because this requires an additional appointment it is unpopular in practice.

The degree of final glaze will also affect the appearance and a high glaze is seldom required. Thus a medium glaze can be accepted as the standard and only exceptions to this noted in the prescription.

Temporary crowns

Temporary crowns are discussed fully in Chapter 4. For anterior teeth the appearance must be adequate and the gingival margin must be maintained in a healthy state.

Temporary crowns are commonly constructed in a rush when time is running out at the end of an appointment and this leads frequently to inadequate construction.

The preferred choice of temporary crown is one that will sit positively on the tooth and have an accurate marginal fit. Time saved by short cuts in temporary crown construction may affect the long-term outcome. The occlusion should be checked carefully before the patient is dismissed and the crown trimmed to avoid any premature contact as this is the commonest cause of discomfort and early loss. Acrylic resin crowns constructed on the study cast in the laboratory are the most satisfactory solution, if the cost is not prohibitive. They do save clinical time and avoid a hasty conclusion to an appointment. However, the alternatives discussed in Chapter 4 are often equally satisfactory.

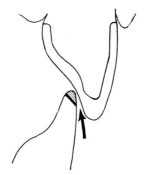

Try-in

The advantages of trying in porcelain crowns at the biscuit bake stage has already been mentioned. This enables some trimming of tight contact points that prevent the crown from being seated and also some adjustment of the length. If a try-in is undertaken at this stage, it is advisable to approach it systematically as follows:

1. Contact points. Overbuilding of the approximal surfaces of the crown is the most common cause of failure to seat the restoration. These contacts are gradually relieved with a carborundum stone used with water to prevent overheating and possible fracture. A length of dental floss may be used for testing the contacts.

   Pressure must never be used to seat a crown because the brittle porcelain may fracture.
2. Peripheral fit. The quality of the fit at the shoulder should be tested with a sharp probe. Any excess of porcelain will be detected and should be removed on the die by the use of a paper-backed carborundum disc or special fine stones which are used at ultra-speeds.
3. Occlusion. The occlusion in centric relation and all excursions of the mandible are checked, using thin articulating paper and occlusal indicator wax, to record any high spots on the crown. These are removed with a carborundum stone or diamond instrument. Slight modification of the opposing incisal edges will reduce many of the adverse stresses (Figure 7.12).
4. Shape and shade. Occasionally, after the crown has been seated it will be found that slight modifications to the shape may be required. Stoning may be done at the chairside but for additions the crown, together with the necessary instructions, will have to be returned to the technician. It should be borne in mind that repeated firings can affect the shade. The patient should at all times be consulted and share in the decision regarding the final appearance of the crown. Minor changes in the shade and characterization of the shape are always possible.

Cementation and finishing

As this stage is usually undertaken without local anaesthesia, it is necessary to warn the patient that some sensation should be expected.

Figure 7.13 (a) Fractured upper central incisors. The upper right central incisor has been root filled and the upper left central incisor has remained vital. (b) Upper right central incisor prepared for cast post and core and the upper left central incisor prepared for a jacket crown. (c) Complete crowns

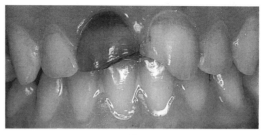

a

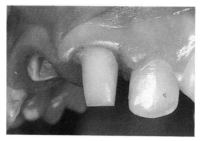

b

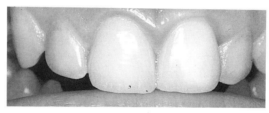

c

Zinc phosphate cement has been used for many decades with excellent results. The pulp of the tooth is less likely to be affected by the acid cement if the temporary crown has been cemented with zinc oxide–eugenol or the tooth is protected by varnish. Some of the zinc oxide–eugenol based cements may also be used for the final cementation. However, many practitioners prefer the water-based glass ionomer cements for the final cementation of the crown.

The tooth and surrounding area of the mouth should be isolated and the preparation dried as for the insertion of a conventional restoration. A fairly thin mix of cement is then placed on all fitting surfaces of the crown, which is gently eased into position on the tooth. It must be well supported by finger and thumb on labial and palatal surfaces, and steady pressure is maintained during the setting time of the cement.

Finishing is usually confined to the removal of excess cement when it has set hard. Any suitable hand instrument can be used to fracture it away cleanly from the margins of the crown.

The periphery of the crown is dried with a jet of warm air. This deflects the free gingivae and allows a visual examination of the margins to be made. Finally, the occlusion is rechecked, and dental floss is used to ensure that all cement debris is removed from the interproximal areas.

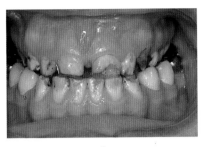

a

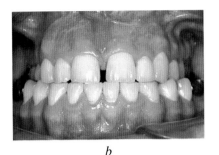

b

Figure 7.14 A young man with defective enamel on all remaining teeth. Metal ceramic crowns were used for the posterior teeth but all twelve anterior teeth were restored with porcelain jacket crowns. (a) Before treatment. (b) After treatment

Porcelain veneers

Veneers of composite resin, acrylics or porcelain can be used to improve the appearance of anterior teeth. Minimal tooth preparation is nearly always necessary, preserving sound tooth structure and minimizing possible adverse effects on the pulp and supporting tissues.

Composite resin veneers are simple to place and require no laboratory facilities. Wear, staining and lengthy chairside time to contour correctly and finish the veneer are problems. They may be very useful as a short-term measure.

Preformed acrylic veneers (Mastique) have been used to mask unsightly teeth, particularly in children but the improvement is less than ideal. Dimensions are significantly increased and they are prone to wear and debonding failure between the acrylic veneer and the composite resin used to cement the restoration in place.

Veneers of porcelain can be produced by a variety of laboratory techniques. The fit surface of the veneer can be etched with hydrofluoric acid or grit blasted to produce a mechanically retentive surface for a composite resin lute. This bond is enhanced by a silane layer, which can be placed by the laboratory or at the chairside and forms a chemical bond between porcelain and resin. Retention to the tooth is mechanical in nature, through conventional acid-etching of enamel.

Indications

Porcelain veneers may be used successfully to mask teeth with intrinsic staining or surface defects caused by tetracycline administration, mild enamel hypoplasia or hypomineralization or fluorosis. Discolored non-vital teeth that otherwise might require post-crowns can be veneered successfully, perhaps following bleaching. Veneers are also useful for the correction of peg-shaped lateral incisor teeth, fractured incisal edges, closing proximal spacing and diastemas. When dramatic changes to the shape of teeth are being considered, it is essential that a diagnostic wax-up on a study cast is first carried out.

To ensure long-term success a high standard of oral hygiene and a low and stable caries rate should be achieved. This is particularly important as the cervical margin of the veneer can often be slightly over-contoured and can exacerbate a pre-existing gingivitis, leading ultimately to gingival recession and exposure of unsightly margins.

In all of these situations a veneer is indicated when, other than the defect to be masked, the tooth is substantially sound and in particular has enamel present on most of the labial surface. The alternative of a porcelain jacket crown must always be considered because in many cases this still offers the better result, especially with severely discolored teeth or if large restorations are present.

Contra-indications

1. Severely rotated or overlapped teeth.
2. Loss of substantial amounts of tooth structure; porcelain jacket crowns may provide a better alternative.
3. Gross loss of labial enamel, for example following acid induced erosion.
4. Occlusal disharmonies, parafunction or severe attrition.
5. Lower incisor teeth. These veneers are more complex to place than uppers and should only be attempted when alternatives are unacceptable. The occlusal forces are less favourable than for upper incisors and the available bonding area considerably less.
6. Severely discolored teeth. Opaque layers of porcelain can be used but these often result in over-contoured labial surfaces and a dull, 'lifeless' appearance to the porcelain. Various opaque cementing resins are also available but their results are somewhat unpredictable and will not mask severe stains. Problems also often result at the cervical margin where discolored tooth still shows because the veneer can only be extended onto the enamel covered surface.

General considerations

Veneers can be constructed to cover teeth without any preparation. This will result in over-contouring and they may be difficult to locate accurately during cementation. Tooth preparation is designed to reduce the enamel by an even amount of about 0.5 mm where the veneer is to be placed. It should extend proximally to just short of the contact point and ideally finish just supragingivally in enamel. The veneer is either extended to, or taken over the incisal tip depending upon the need to rebuild this area.

Local anaesthesia is not normally required as the reduction must be kept within enamel. This will also help to ensure that enamel perforation does not take place.

The presence of small proximal restorations does not contra-indicate the use of veneers and they may be incorporated into the preparation. Ideally they should be replaced before veneering to ensure complete caries removal and a good marginal seal. Restoration with a glass–ionomer cement rather than a composite resin will allow for useful bonding to take place between the restoration and the composite lute used for the veneer.

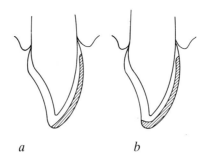

Figure 7.15 Examples of preparation types. (a) Incisal bevel preparation. (b) Overlap incisal preparation

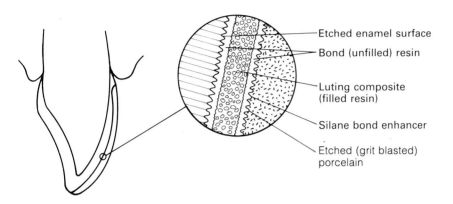

Etched enamel surface

Bond (unfilled) resin

Luting composite (filled resin)

Silane bond enhancer

Etched (grit blasted) porcelain

Figure 7.16 Section through a cemented veneer shows the build-up of layers required for bonding

Several alternative preparations for the incisal edge have been described but only two types are worth considering:

1. The incisal bevel/chamfer preparation (Figure 7.15a). This is the preparation of choice when the tooth being veneered is of the required length. It is obviously better not to remove the tip unless necessary because this makes the preparation more conservative and does not alter the patient's natural incisal guidance and tooth contacts. A bevel is placed at the tip to give an adequate bulk of porcelain at the margin and so prevent chipping of the porcelain. It will also aid seating.
2. Overlapped incisal edge preparation (Figure 7.15b). To be used when it is necessary to lengthen the tooth or to protect part of the palatal surface.

Tooth preparation

Preparation is carried out using water-cooled high speed diamond burs. Initial depth orientation cuts are placed to ensure the correct amount of tooth reduction. A 1 mm diameter round diamond bur is used to dimple the labial surface. If it is used with the bur in the long axis of the tooth, hemi-spherical dimples will be cut to 0.5 mm in depth before the shank prevents deeper cutting (Figure 7.17b). Using a round ended tapered diamond bur the preparation is then continued until the dimples are just removed. A confluent, chamfered finishing line is established proximally and gingivally (Figure 7.17c). Great care must be taken gingivally to prevent perforation of the enamel in this area where it becomes thin. Although small

Figure 7.17 (a) Patient with severe discoloration requiring veneers. (b) Close up of initial preparation using a round diamond bur to place depth cuts. (c) Close up of completed preparations. (d) Porcelain veneers cemented. The |3 was restored with a metal–ceramic crown due to the large restoration already present

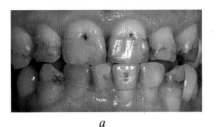

a

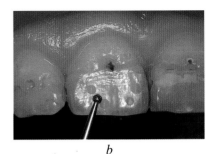

b

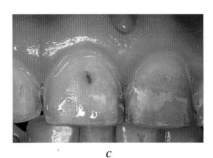

c

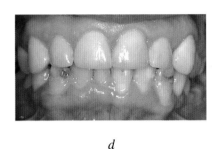

d

areas of the preparation can extend into dentine without adversely affecting retention, it is best to avoid this if at all possible. Dentine bonding agents can be used to bond the resin lute to dentine but this is not ideal, particularly at the margins.

Although it is important that no undercut areas are produced in the preparation, care should be taken to ensure that the veneer extends adequately in the proximal areas adjacent to the gingival papilla. An unsightly band of uncovered tooth will show, especially when viewed from the side, unless this area is included in the preparation. A labial rather than an incisal path of insertion should be prepared. (The incisal edge is dealt with as described (Figure 7.15).)

The surface produced with conventional coarse diamond burs is adequate for the preparation as bonding with composite resins will be facilitated by the rough surface. A finishing bur may be used to refine the margins.

When dealing with a tooth to be built out by the veneer, such as a peg shaped lateral incisor, it is still advantageous to carry out some tooth preparation to improve the bond and gingival contour. A fine, chamfered margin should be produced but it is not necessary to reduce the tooth by a full 0.5 mm. Alternatively, a severely discolored tooth or a rotated tooth, can benefit from deeper preparation in areas as long as the enamel is not lost at the margins.

Impression

An impression is taken using any of the elastomeric materials. Stock trays can be used, but it is useful to place stops on teeth away from those prepared to stop penetration of the incisal edges through the impression material onto the tray itself. As a general rule it is useful to take a full arch impression to allow for a full articulation with an opposing cast. Only if the veneers are completely confined to the labial surface and will not come into contact with opposing teeth can a part arch impression be used. This must include adjacent teeth to demonstate required tooth contours.

Retraction cord is rarely necessary and if required is often a sign of over-preparation. Simple blowing with an air syringe should reveal the margin and allow access for a low viscosity material to record its detail.

Shade selection, details for characterization and the need for opaque porcelain to mask out severe discolorations should all be noted.

Temporary coverage

This is seldom required as the appearance of the prepared teeth has not been altered significantly and there is likely to be only very mild sensitivity to cold or hot. It is essential that the patient maintains ideal plaque control at this stage so that cementation can take place with healthy marginal gingivae.

If pre-existing failed veneers are being replaced, the patient may request temporary veneers to prevent disclosure of teeth with a poor appearance between preparation and cementation. In this instance composite resin may be placed over the preparations, but it should not be bonded into place using acid-etching of the enamel as this will make subsequent removal and bonding of the final veneer less accurate. Composite resin should adhere adequately to dry enamel without etching.

Laboratory techniques

Laboratory techniques are outside the remit of this book. However, the reader should be aware of the processes involved. Several techniques are in common use:

1. Using refractory dies that are able to withstand the high temperatures required to fuse porcelain.
2. Using platinum foil adapted to a die in a similar manner to the production of porcelain jacket crowns.
3. Using castable ceramic techniques.

Following construction the fit surface is roughened either using hydrofluoric acid or by grit blasting with 50 μm aluminium oxide particles.

To enhance the bond between resin and porcelain, the veneers may be treated with a silane bonding agent. These bond to silica within the porcelain and have a free methacrylate group that bonds to the composite resin. Although they do contribute a chemical bond between the two materials this is not as significant as the mechanical linkage already achieved.

If a silane layer has been used, care must be taken not to contaminate this during the try-in stage and several chairside bonding kits provide a silane solution to be applied immediately before veneer insertion.

Try-in

The prepared teeth are first cleaned with a slurry of pumice and water, then dried. Isolation with cotton wool rolls, suction and gauze to protect the airway are used while individual veneer fit and contour are checked. If multiple veneers are being placed they should then be tried-in together to check that contact areas are not overbuilt. Care must be taken not to seat the veneer too forcefully. Adjustment with fine diamond burs is possible but the veneers are fragile at this stage and minor adjustment is often best left until it is bonded into place.

The shade of luting resin should now be chosen. Composite resin cements with a low viscosity are used, and these are normally light cured. Dual cured resins may be necessary if the veneer is very opaque. A cement with a water-soluble try-in paste is used under the veneer to assess which shade is required. Alternatively the actual cement can be used by turning off the operating light, placing a small amount of the composite onto the fit surface of the veneer, which has been previously wetted with water, and seating this onto the tooth, which has also been moistened. The shade can then be quickly assessed, the veneer removed and excess resin wiped with cotton wool. The veneer should then be placed in acetone to dissolve any remaining resin. Excess cement should also be removed from the tooth quickly. Different shades may be tried until the desired effect is achieved. There is little scope for the operator to significantly alter the shade of the veneer.

Opaque resins are available to mask heavily pigmented areas. If this is required, it is normally necessary to remove further tooth structure in that area to make room for the resin.

Following try-in, the fit surface of the veneer should be cleaned, dried and re-coated with the silane bonding agent.

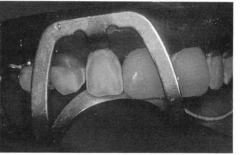

a

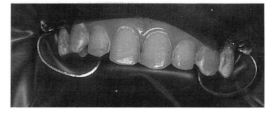

b

Figure 7.18 Isolation during cementation. (a) With a full rubber dam retracted by a clamp. (b) Alternatively, using a split dam

Cementation

The isolation of the tooth should now be considered. Ideally a rubber dam is used to isolate the tooth. This can be very difficult to retract into the sulcus sufficiently and may hinder cementation (Figure 7.18). Strict control with cotton wool rolls, saliva ejectors and sponges must be used. It is essential that damage is not caused to the gingival tissues to avoid bleeding. Gingival retraction cord may be used to limit this problem.

Adjacent teeth are protected by placement of a soft metal matrix or a mylar matrix strip (Figure 7.19a). This can be held in place with proximal wedges.

The tooth is acid-etched in the conventional manner for 30 seconds, washed for 20 seconds and dried with oil-free air until a frosted appearance is evident. A layer of unfilled bonding resin is applied, blown with air to ensure that it is as thin as possible and cured. If areas of exposed dentine are present, a dentine bonding agent should be used according to the manufacturer's instructions.

The chosen composite is then placed as a thin layer in the veneer, care being taken not to incorporate any air bubbles. Without touching the resin, the veneer is carefully seated onto the tooth incisally first, with a slight 'jiggling' motion to ensure that it is fully seated. With a probe or a brush dipped in unfilled resin, gross excess cement is removed from the margins. If the position of the veneer is correct, it is first tacked into place with a 10-second cure from the light in the tip area. Further removal of excess is possible, but care must be taken not to drag out the cement from under the margins. Curing of the composite can then be completed by directing the light on the incisal, labial and proximal areas for at least 60 seconds.

Adjacent veneers can then be cemented in a similar manner, one at a time.

Finishing

Gross excess cement can be chipped off with hand instruments, such as scalers; remaining excess cement is carefully removed from the margins with water-cooled fine diamond burs. These can also be used to trim porcelain margins finely. Proximal areas are finished with composite polishing strips to ensure that floss passes easily through the contact. Final polishing of the margins is achieved with impregnated polishing points, polishing pastes or composite polishing discs.

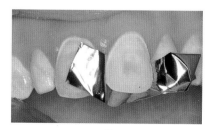

a

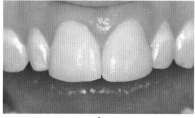

b

Figure 7.19 (a) Prepared incisor teeth with soft metal foil in place. The |1 has been acid etched. (b) Completed veneers

Occlusal contacts are checked to ensure that there is no excessive contact on the veneer in intercuspal position or any occlusal excursion.

As it is often difficult to ensure complete removal of excess cement at this visit, it is essential that the patient is seen again one week later for final finishing and to check that the correct oral hygiene techniques are being employed.

Maintenance

At regular follow-up appointments, marginal integrity and signs of leakage, colour and aesthetic stability and gingival health should be checked. Properly executed veneers rarely fail due to bonding failure. They are highly successful conservative restorations. Patients engaged in contact sports should be provided with a mouth guard made in the laboratory.

Metal–ceramic crowns

The metal–ceramic crown is a full veneer that can be used in either the anterior or posterior region of the mouth. It is a metal alloy that has dental porcelain bonded onto either all or most of its surfaces. It is strong and versatile. It can be constructed to have the palatal surface in a very thin section to accommodate the opposing teeth. It can be soldered to other retainers of a bridge and to pontics. However, it requires much tooth reduction of the labial surface where porcelain has to be added.

Indications:

1. As a single unit in the anterior region. However, it is often difficult to obtain a good appearance because of the need to mask the metal framework.
2. Where, in view of the brittleness of the material, a porcelain jacket crown is not indicated. In such situations the stronger metal ceramic crown has its place.
3. When minimal inter-occlusal space is available.
4. When strength and maximum resistance to occlusal forces is required.

Contra-indications:

1. When the need for much tooth reduction might endanger the pulp.
2. When it is impossible to obtain a good appearance cervically because of the metal framework. In such situations it is often necessary to use shoulder porcelain to avoid a grey gingival margin (see Figure 8.10b).

The material

Metal–ceramic restorations were developed to overcome the brittleness of all-porcelain crowns. All-porcelain jacket crowns rely on a minimum thickness of porcelain of 0.8 mm to resist the forces of occlusion or mastication. Therefore in many cases, such as high parafunctional loads or bruxism, all-porcelain crowns are contra-indicated. The ability to bond porcelain to metal has provided an alternative crown for use where appearance is important. The gold alloys contain approximately 80% gold and from 6% to 15% platinum, so that the cost of the material is obviously important.

Gold–platinum–palladium alloys are widely used. One disadvantage is that their melting point is rather close to the fusing temperature of the porcelains used (900–950°C). This gives them the tendency to 'creep' during firing of the porcelain, which may affect the marginal fit of the restoration, especially with large castings such as bridges. Careful design of the metal at the cervical margin may help to prevent lifting away from the preparation of a thin metal margin when the porcelain is fused. Thus a distinct chamfered margin will offer less resistance to creep than a rounded margin.

When the appearance of the metal is important, a non-palladium alloy containing tantalum may be used. This has the traditional appearance of gold and minimizes the risk of hydrogen porosity within the porcelain. Gold–palladium–silver alloys have higher melting points, which avoid the problems of creep during firing of the porcelain. Because of the 50% gold content and the lack of platinum they are considerably cheaper than the high-gold alloys.

It is difficult to obtain a satisfactory fit consistently with palladium–silver alloys. They also possess all the disadvantages of other alloys containing palladium and silver.

Non-precious metal alloys are based on nickel and chromium or cobalt and chromium. The bond between the alloy casting and porcelain can be good but the oxides of chromium and nickel can affect not only the bond strength but also the appearance of the bonded facing. Chromium can reduce oxides in the porcelain giving a grey colour with the reduction products.

Clinical considerations

A layer of both metal and porcelain must be accommodated on the labial surface of the tooth that is to be restored with a metal ceramic crown. The effect of providing this space must be assessed at the planning stage. A thickness of 1.5 mm is needed to accommodate the two materials and also allow the translucency required for a good appearance. Therefore, extensive tooth reduction might endanger the pulp or weaken the tooth, in which case an alternative type of crown should be considered.

The preparation has to provide support for the porcelain to prevent cohesive fracture within it. Unsupported porcelain is unable to cope with high-tensile stresses, which can originate at the occlusal junction of porcelain and alloy.

An intra-porcelain fracture due to cohesive failure seldom affects the integrity of the crown. Nevertheless, it may necessitate replacement because of poor appearance. Sometimes a very special type of repair may be carried out and this is described in Chapter 11.

With anterior metal–ceramic crowns it is difficult to obtain good appearance of the labial margins of the restoration as well as good strength.

Figure 7.20 (a) Labial shoulder margin design with metal substructure finishing short of margin to allow a porcelain butt joint for optimum appearance. (b) Chamfer margin suitable for preparations on teeth with gingival recession when the preparation is extended past the enamel margin onto the root. This type of metal margin alloows good appearance while keeping the preparation conservative in design. (c) The bevelled shoulder preparation design produces a metal collar, which gives maximum resistance to creep and makes it easier for the technician to produce a precise marginal fit. It can only be used when the margin is hidden by the upper lip

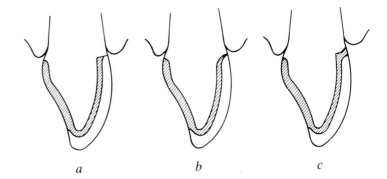

a   *b*   *c*

Careful design is necessary to avoid a thick labial margin placed to mask the underlying metal. There are several basic labial finishing lines. For anterior metal ceramic crowns a labial shoulder is usually the preferred design. However, the bevelled shoulder produces the least distortion during the firing of the crown (Figure 7.20).

Alternatively, a full 90° shoulder may be used and the metal can be brought out to the margin or left short of the margin for a better appearance. The porcelain margin is the design of choice when the patient retracts the lip during speech to expose the cervical margins of the crown (Figure 7.21).

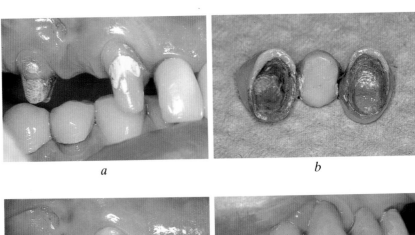

a   *b*

Figure 7.21 (a) Canine and second premolar prepared for a metal ceramic bridge. On smiling, the patient will expose the margins of both abutments. (b) The porcelain margins of both retainers. (c) The fitted metal ceramic bridge with good marginal appearance. (d) A similar metal ceramic bridge in another patient with a porcelain margin only on the anterior (canine) retainer. The metal is clearly visible on the second (premolar) retainer. The patient could not expose the margin of this tooth during speech or when smiling

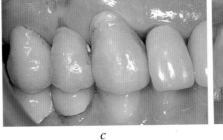
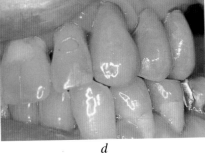

c   *d*

The preparation

The essential features of the preparation of an anterior tooth for a metal–ceramic crown are similar to those for a porcelain jacket crown. However, there are some fundamental differences:

1. Labially, the reduction of the tooth must be sufficient to accommodate the metal, the opaque layer of porcelain to mask the metal and the translucent porcelain. For this the ideal amount of reduction is 2 mm, although most operators would accept 1.5 mm as adequate. This is one of the essential features of the preparation because less than 1.5 mm reduction will result in either a poor, lifeless appearance or an overbuilding of the porcelain facing in an effort to mask the opaque layer and metal. This usually makes the contour of the crown quite unacceptable.
2. The labial cervical margin can be in porcelain or metal depending on the appearance required. Many patients do not expose their cervical margins during normal speech and it is advisable to discuss with the patient the advantages and disadvantages of placing the margin of the crown subgingivally.

    When there is no need for a subgingival margin, it is much healthier for the gingivae to finish the preparation either level with the soft tissues or supragingivally.

    It is obvious that subgingival margins initially tend to result in a better appearance but there is always the risk of gingival inflammation or recession, which will not be apparent for some weeks or months.
3. Interproximally and palatally the margins can be finished to a chamfer and only minimal reduction of the tooth is required to accommodate the thickness of the metal. Generally 0.5 mm reduction is adequate.

    The extension of porcelain on the palatal surface of the crown depends on the occlusion and the need to have occlusal contact with either metal or porcelain, but not both.

Post retained crowns

When there is insufficient coronal tooth structure to retain a simple crown many different techniques are possible to increase retention; one example is a post crown (Figure 7.22). A post crown derives retention from a metal post cemented into the prepared root canal with a core attached, over which the crown is cemented (Figure 7.23). This commonly follows root canal therapy when much dentine may have been lost following caries or trauma, and access has been made for endodontics. To place a crown on a non-vital tooth weakened internally by endodontic preparation and externally by crown preparation is to risk fracture of the complete clinical crown.

Not all root filled teeth that require crowns need to have posts placed. Root filled teeth are weaker than vital teeth. The amount of remaining dentine following crown preparation must be assessed in each case. For example, a pinned amalgam core may be adequate in a molar tooth, see Chapter 8.

Figure 7.22 2| restored with a post crown, (a) on presentation, (b) post and core in place and (c) completed porcelain crown

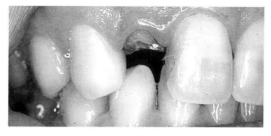

a

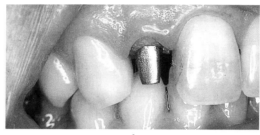

b

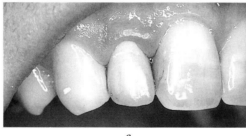

c

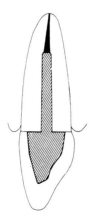

Figure 7.23 Crown, post and core *in situ*

The placement of a post should be considered as an aid to retention for the crown, not as a method of reinforcing the root. In fact a post can considerably weaken the root if dentine is unnecessarily removed during its preparation.

Post retained crowns are one of the most difficult restorations to produce reliably and tend to have a high failure rate, particularly due to lack of retention. For this reason, many techniques exist to minimize this problem.

Clinical assessment of the individual tooth

The factors to be considered in assessing a tooth for a post crown are similar to those already discussed in Chapter 1. Some elaboration of the radiographic investigation, however, is necessary. Special attention must be given to the following:

1. Length of the root. It appears that on an empirical basis it would seem wise to have a length of post within the root as long as possible leaving a minimum of 3 to 4 mm remaining root canal filling to ensure that there is no leakage from the apical seal. Where the root has been shortened by apicectomy, resorption, caries or fracture, some modification of the normal post preparation may be necessary to compensate for the loss of post length. The alternative solutions are discussed later in the chapter.
2. Alignment of the root. The line of withdrawal of the post impression will be dictated by the direction of the root canal. Any abnormality in relation to adjacent teeth may affect the withdrawal of impressions and the fitting of a crown.
3. Quality of the root filling. The root filling should be well condensed gutta percha, especially in the apical third of the root canal (Figure 7.24).

    Sometimes a radiograph may show an inadequate root filling but no evidence of a canal beyond it and no evidence of periapical infection. Such a tooth, in the absence of clinical symptoms, may be regarded as suitable for a post crown without further endodontic treatment. If a new root canal filling has been placed it is best to wait at least 3 months to

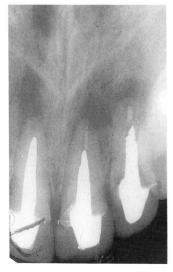

a

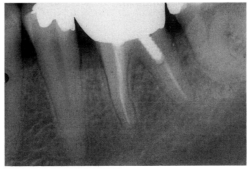

b

Figure 7.24 (a) Post placed in the absence of adequate root canal fillings with consequent periapical radiolucencies. (b) Well root-treated molar tooth with a post retained crown in place

ensure success before placing a post in the canal. There are many situations where this is not practical, for instance, if an anterior crown is missing, the post has to be placed immediately.

On the other hand, a radiograph may reveal evidence of a periapical condition that necessitates an apicectomy. It is normal to place the new post in the canal before the apicectomy is performed.

Risks

Restoring a tooth with a post crown is an extreme decision taken with the knowledge that this restoration has a high failure rate. The following are the most likely risks:

1. Root fracture. The root canal space required for a post of adequate strength may weaken the root and lead to its fracture.
2. Root perforation. During the preparation of the post-hole there is a risk of perforating the root and thereby jeopardizing the entire restoration.
3. Loss of post. Even well-fitting cast or pre-formed posts may become loose with time. The cement seal appears to be especially vulnerable to torsional stress or repeated axial stress. Therefore, the post should not be circular in cross-section for the whole of its length and great care must be taken to remove occlusal interferences.
4. Corrosion. The junction between two dissimilar metals will cause corrosion and this is demonstrated when a gold core is cast onto a nickel–chrome post.

There is no consensus of opinion about an optimal post-crown design or type for this high-risk restoration, and at present there are many options. A representative selection of these is discussed in the following pages.

Types available

The confusing range of techniques available can be simplified by consideration of the following features of post design:

Manufacture: ready made/custom made.
Post shape: tapered/parallel.
Post surface: smooth/serrated/threaded.
Components: post and core, and separate crown/one-piece post crown.
Material: precious metal/non-precious metal.

All techniques are a mixture of these design features. The most successful and commonly used techniques are:

1. Parallel-sided cast post and cores, produced using preformed impression templates matched to twist drills and laboratory casting patterns (Parapost: Whaledent; Op-op post, Optident, UK).
2. Ready-made parallel posts used in conjunction with a plastic restorative material for the core (Parapost: Whaledent; Op-op post, Optident, UK).
3. Tapered custom-made cast post and cores produced freehand or utilizing preformed impression templates (Produit-Dentaire: P.D.).

4. Ready-made parallel-sided threaded posts and plastic cores (Radix Ankor, Maillefer, France; Kurer crown saver, Cottrell, London; Flexipost, Svedia, Sweden).

Design features

Length of the post
The longer the post that is placed, the greater the retention. This is limited by:

1. The need to retain a minimum of 3 to 4 mm of undisturbed root filling at the apex.
2. The risk of over-preparation of the apical end of the post-hole and possible perforation if a parallel post is used with a diameter suitable for a snug fit coronally.

As a general rule the post should be at least as long as the crown it will retain. Ideally it will utilize the entire length available as determined by an accurate long-cone periapical radiograph.

Parallel vs. tapered designs
Parallel-sided posts offer significant increases in retention over tapered posts of the same length. Root canals are, however, tapered in shape and this may be exaggerated if caries has destroyed dentine in the coronal opening. A tapered post-hole would overcome this problem of differing diameters but would thereby lose valuable retention. There is usually some part of the root canal that can be prepared with parallel sides without perforating the root.

Diameter of the post
It is unwise to use the extreme coronal section of the root canal to gauge the width of the proposed post-hole. This part of the canal is seldom circular in cross-section and any attempt to make it so could result in too large a post-hole. The irregular shape will, in any case, assist resistance form and prevent rotation.

To prevent the risk of the post bending under load, it should have a minimum cross-sectional diameter of 1.5 mm at the coronal opening. The use of stronger non-precious metal posts can overcome the problem of bending. A compromise must sometimes be accepted between the strength of the post and the strength of the remaining root, for example in lower incisor teeth.

Surface configuration of the post
Custom-made cast posts normally have a smooth finish and can be made more retentive by sand blasting. Pre-formed post systems often offer significant advantages for retention, as post surfaces can be serrated (Figure 7.25) or even threaded. Threaded posts derive retention by engaging dentine, and dramatically increase the retention for a post of a given length,

Figure 7.25 Parallel-sided cast
post (Parapost) showing the
ribbed surface and cement release
channel

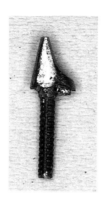

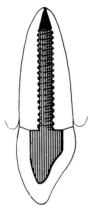

Figure 7.26 The Kurer anchor.
The threaded post is cemented
into the prepared canal

but care must be taken to avoid over-stressing the root during preparation
and cementation (Figure 7.26).

Material for the post
Conventional casting gold may well not be adequate to resist bending unless
used in thick section. Therefore, non-precious metals or wrought precious
metal can be used. Problems have arisen in the past with an increased risk of
root fracture, leakage and root discoloration when base metals have been
used, particularly when combined with cast gold cores. It is essential to use
similar metals for the posts and cores.

Separate or one-piece post-crowns
One-piece post-crowns are normally only used when there is insufficient
space to make a retentive core for a separate crown. For example if there has
been loss of inter-alveolar space due to attrition of the natural crowns and
compensating over-eruption or with short clinical crowns.

Resistance form
Consideration must be given to the design of the post to prevent functional
loads from causing dislodgment. To prevent the post being circular in
cross-section an anti-rotation slot is placed in the region where most residual
thickness of dentine remains. Residual dentine on the coronal root face
should be sound and ideally at right angles to the loads likely to be faced.

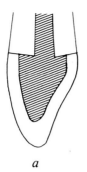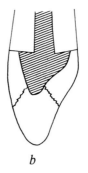

a   *b*

Figure 7.27 The core shown in (a) allows a uniform thickness of porcelain, which is strong. The core shown in (b) requires an excess bulk of porcelain incisally, which is liable to fracture across the labial or palatal face. There is also less retention and resistance to displacement in (b) than in (a)

Core design
The core can be shaped to provide ideal retention for the crown and allow optimum thickness for the restoration (Figure 7.27). It will follow the basic shape that the tooth would have had if it had been intact and prepared as described in the relevant chapter.

Choice of type of post and core

Anterior teeth
Five techniques are suitable, all of which have their advantages and disadvantages.

Custom made tapered cast post and core (Figure 7.28)
Advantages:

1. Universal technique possible for any shaped canal.
2. Follows the canal shape, so unlikely to weaken or perforate the canal.
3. Defects in the coronal dentine can be filled in with the casting and a diaphragm can be incorporated if required.

Disadvantages:

1. Less retentive than other posts, therefore need to be of optimum length.
2. Cannot utilize wrought metals.
3. Temporary post-crowns are complex to make and retain.
4. Impression techniques are complex.
5. Laboratory work involved.

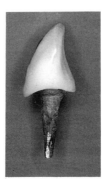

Figure 7.28 Freehand cast tapered post with crown attached

Figure 7.29 The various components of a Parapost kit. The post bur is matched by (from the left) a steel post to be used for a direct build up, a laboratory burn out post, a plastic impression post and (on the right) an aluminium temporary post

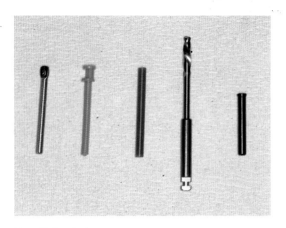

Parallel-sided cast   *re using pre-formed kit* (Figure 7.29)
Advantages:

1. Adaptable technique allowing for any shaped coronal canal with a precisely fitting apical portion.
2. Highly retentive.
3. Temporary crowns and impressions simplified by pre-formed components.
4. Serrations possible on post surface to improve retention.
5. Any metal can be used for the casting.

Disadvantages:

1. Less retentive than threaded posts.
2. Care must be taken not to over-prepare the apical portion.
3. Laboratory work involved.

Tapered cast post and core using pre-formed kit
As for parallel-sided cast post and core using pre-formed kit, but less retentive.

Parallel-sided ready-made post and plastic core (Figure 7.30)
Advantages:

1. Does not require a laboratory stage or a temporary post.
2. Non-precious metals can be used.

Disadvantages:

1. Longer clinical procedure.
2. The crown margin needs to extend 1 mm or more beyond the core material. The technique is, therefore, not suitable if the bulk of the coronal structure has been lost.

Threaded post and plastic core (Figure 7.31)
Advantages:

1. Highly retentive therefore suitable for short roots.

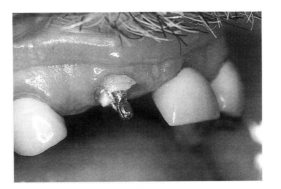

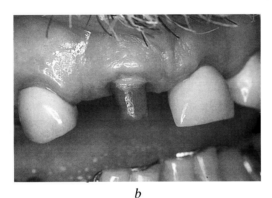

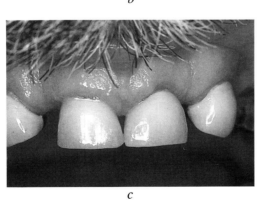

Figure 7.30 Direct core build up using composite. (a) Stainless steel parapost and dentine pin in place. (b) Coloured composite core cured and shaped. (c) Complete crown (note the labial margin is a poor fit)

Disadvantages:

1. Great care should be taken to prepare the root canal correctly and cement the post without exerting undue stress on the remaining dentine.

Note. Tapered threaded posts are not recommended because they cut their own threads on insertion and so exert considerable stress on the dentine.

For anterior teeth the authors prefer to use cast parallel-sided posts using a pre-formed system for preparation, impression taking and production, rather than building up a plastic core in the mouth.

Figure 7.31 Radix Ankors

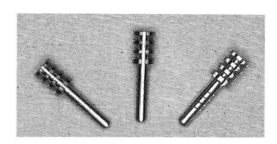

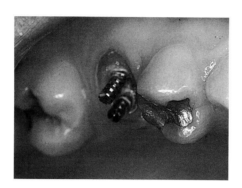

Figure 7.32 Two flexi-posts in place utilizing both canals in an upper premolar tooth ready for core build up

Posterior teeth
1. Pinned core. Suitable if sufficient coronal dentine remains, see Chapter 8.
2. Ready made post and plastic core (Figure 7.32). Posts may be passively fitting or threaded, and can utilize one or more canals. Accessory dentine pins can be used to aid retention.
3. Custom-made cast post and cores. Can be made either in one piece using one canal or two if the canals can be prepared parallel (perhaps with the second canal shorter) or as a two-piece casting that locks together in the core.

Due to the complexity of manufacturing techniques 1 or 2 are recommended rather than 3. The authors prefer to use pre-formed parallel-sided, non-precious metal posts to retain an amalgam core for root-filled posterior teeth where substantial coronal structure has been lost.

Preparation

The basic stages are applicable to all types of post and core and are as follows.

Stage 1
The remaining coronal dentine for the crown is prepared placing the margin as required and reducing the clinical portion of the tooth by half. The preparation can be more generous than normal for a crown on a vital tooth; however, as much as practical coronal dentine should be retained (Figure 7.33).

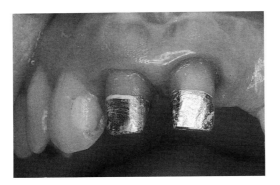

Figure 7.33 Gold post and cores in place showing the retention of a maximum amount of coronal dentine. The core is used solely to replace the missing structure

Stage 2

Having assessed the likely possible length and width of the post from the radiograph, the root filling is removed to the required level.

Several methods are available to remove gutta percha, which is easiest to achieve without disturbing the apical seal if the gutta percha has been well-condensed. Gates Glidden drills are most suitable for this and should be run at low speed because any heat generated will cause it to stick to the drill. Rose head burs with a long shank can also be used at slow speed, care being taken to follow the canal. A size should be chosen that is just wider than the gutta percha point to be removed. Alternatively, twist drills can be used, but these also can perforate through the side of the canal so they must be used with great care.

It is also possible to remove gutta percha with hot instruments carefully inserted into the canal. However, it is unlikely that these can be introduced far enough down the canal to be entirely effective.

Solvents are not recommended for removal of gutta percha because their spread is not easy to control.

If a silver point is present in the canal then it is best to remove this first and replace it with a good gutta percha filling.

Some cements may be very hard to remove and if there is any doubt as to the orientation of the canal it is far better to stop, examine the preparation carefully and perhaps take a check radiograph to re-orientate, rather than risk perforation.

Stage 3

The post-hole is shaped either using tapered or parallel-sided burs as required. It is better to start off with smaller diameter burs and increase in size until the required diameter is reached.

Stage 4

An anti-rotation groove may be required.

Stage 5

Any remaining weakened dentine (less than 1 mm in thickness) left between the shoulder and the post-hole is removed and sharp corners are rounded off.

Impressions

The impression technique chosen for post crowns is dependent upon the method chosen for post construction. Use of a parallel-sided pre-formed post avoids the very difficult task of securing an accurate impression of the entire post-hole as it is impossible to take a satisfactory impression of a parallel-sided post-hole. Alternative impression techniques are described for the various techniques:

1. Indirect technique for use with pre-formed cast posts (parallel or tapered). The plastic impression post from the kit should be tried-in and checked to ensure it reaches to the end of the preparation and is a tight fit. The coronal end should be cut off so that it extends into the body of the impression material but does not touch the tray, flattened out with a hot instrument and coated with adhesive.

   The impression is then taken in the conventional way using an elastomeric material. The post is first inserted in the canal and impression material syringed into the coronal opening to record the anti-rotation lock and the remaining root face.

   On withdrawal from the mouth it should be checked to ensure that the post is firmly held within the impression (Figure 7.34).

2. Indirect impression technique. Suitable for a tapered cast post and core. It is possible to take one impression including the post preparation if the post-section is reinforced with a wire that extends from the apical end of the preparation well into the body of the impression. With care the exact relationships of post-hole, root preparation and adjacent teeth can be preserved in the cast.

   The stages are as follows: (a) A strong piece of wire that will fit loosely within the canal and reach the apical end is required. The coronal part of this roughened wire is looped to lock into the body of the impression but not impinge upon the tray. (b) A syringe or tube is required with a nozzle fine enough to reach as near as possible to the apex of the post canal. This is filled with mixed elastic impression material (light-bodied) and inserted into the canal. The impression material will extrude as the nozzle is gradually withdrawn. The wire, which has been coated with adhesive, is immediately inserted into the entire length of the canal. (c) The

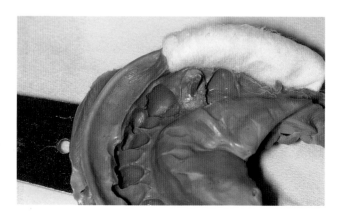

Figure 7.34 Impression of post preparations using matched plastic impression posts

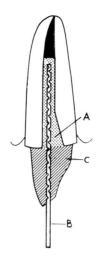

Figure 7.35 The direct impression for a post and core. Inlay wax (A) supported by wire (B), which is sufficiently long to act as a sprue. (C) Core formed in wax or resin

remaining mixed impression material is syringed around the rest of the preparation and the wire loop, and the filled tray is seated.

After withdrawal, the impression is examined for air-blows in the post-hole. Small defects can be blocked out in the laboratory.

3. Direct impression for a cast post and core (pre-formed or freehand). A direct pattern for a post and core can offer greater control by eliminating one stage of the laboratory procedure. However, it does take more chairside time. If a pre-formed post pattern is to be used, this is trimmed as above and the core formed in wax or an acrylic such as Duralay. Alternatively, a direct pattern of the post-hole for a tapered post can be produced using wax on a roughened wire in a lightly lubricated canal (Figure 7.35).

The opposing teeth
A full impression of the opposing teeth is taken in alginate. The model should be cast immediately ready for use in assessing the occlusion during construction of the core and the subsequent crown. Jaw relationship records are also taken if required, see Chapter 3.

Temporary restoration

Pre-formed post kits include a temporary post to fit in the prepared canal accurately. These can be made of aluminium or titanium and are incorporated into an acrylic or resin provisional crown, produced as described in Chapter 4. If a tapered cast post that is not pre-formed is used, a temporary wire post can be incorporated into a conventional temporary crown (Figure 7.36). It is not wise to let the material flow down the post-hole, and therefore cotton wool is first wrapped around the end of the wire and inserted into the canal. The temporary crown is then manufactured and acrylic material allowed to extend into the coronal half of the post-hole.

When the temporary post is cemented a temporary cement is used, coating only the coronal half of the post, so that cement is not introduced into the apical end of the post-hole.

Figure 7.36 Temporary post crown using a pre-formed post and polycarbonate crown former. A clinical example is seen in Figure 4.2

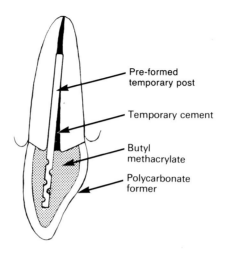

Pre-formed temporary post

Temporary cement

Butyl methacrylate

Polycarbonate former

Try-in

The try-in routine should be similar to that described in Chapter 6. An occasional complication with post crowns, however, deserves special mention. If the impression of the root canal is slightly distorted during withdrawal, the resulting casting may be slightly elongated and cause difficulty in seating the post and core. Reduction of the length of the post by a small amount usually overcomes this complication. The use of pre-formed patterns avoids the problem.

Cementation

The tooth must be isolated, and the prepared face and post-hole dried thoroughly. If the post and core, and crown, have been produced together, they should be cemented with the same thin mix of cement. Alternatively, the post and core is cemented and then a further impression is taken for the crown. Any of the cements commonly used for cementation are used (see Chapter 6).

A thin mix is inserted into the post-hole using an endodontic file rotated anticlockwise, coating the walls of the post-hole with cement. The post and gingival base of the core are coated with cement and inserted into the canal with firm pressure. It is essential that continued pressure is used until the cement is set because with a firmly fitting post considerable hydrostatic pressure can occur within the canal, and the post will rise up out of the canal if not firmly held in place. The pre-formed posts usually have a channel incorporated within the post to vent the excess cement and ensure complete seating within the canal. The excess cement is removed when set hard.

Special problems

1. The apicectomized tooth. Many teeth require post crowns following root filling and apicectomy (Figure 7.37). It is normally best to place the post before the apicectomy so that there is no chance of the retrograde root filling being displaced during cementation of the post.

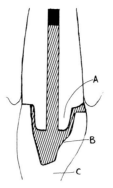

Figure 7.37 A post crown on an apicectomized tooth showing the dentine stump (A) supported by a cast-gold 'thimble' and post (B) with a porcelain jacket crown (C) cemented to it. Note the level of the palatal margin

Particular problems exist if the remaining tooth is not long enough to offer support for a conventional post. A threaded post can be considered in this instance as it will offer significantly greater retention over a conventional post. Great care must be taken during preparation and insertion of these posts to avoid overstressing the remaining root and inducing root fracture.

2. The malpositioned tooth. Sometimes an instanding or protruding tooth may make it impossible to construct the core and crown in the same plane as the root. It is possible to angle the post and core up to 30° as shown in Figure 7.38a.

A similar procedure may be used to overcome the problems of crowning overlapped teeth (Figure 7.38b) if sufficient space is available between the adjacent teeth to avoid a poor appearance. The problem which remains, however, is one of insufficient space and the best solution is usually obtained by orthodontic treatment. Crowning or elective root treatment followed by post crowns, is not a suitable alternative to the orthodontic treatment of developmental malpositions of teeth where there is insufficient space.

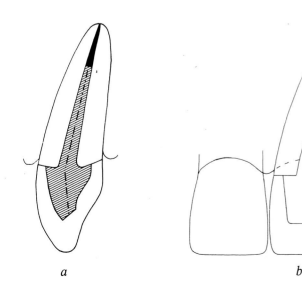

a

b

Figure 7.38 (a) A post crown for a malpositioned tooth showing the post fitted in alignment with the root but with the gold core and jacket crown retruded to reduce the protrusion. (b) A post crown for an overlapping tooth showing the post fitted in alignment with the root, but with the core constructed to give an incisal line of insertion for the jacket crown

Figure 7.39 A post crown showing modification of the core to fill a proximal cavity from which caries or an old filling may have been removed

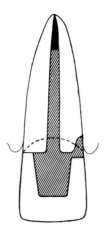

These techniques are only suitable with cast posts as they allow the position of the core to be determined accurately on the models in the laboratory.

3. Subgingival extension. From time to time it will be found that caries or a large restoration will have extended beyond the gingival margin. Also a fracture line may extend subgingivally, which is common palatally on upper incisors. The method of dealing with this is the incorporation of a diaphragm in the cast post and core. This is illustrated in Figure 7.39. Gingivoplasty is often required in order to reveal the gingival margin of the defect. The diaphragm will impart extra stability to the remaining root as well as reduce the chance of root fracture (Figure 7.40). It may be necessary to limit extension of the metal towards the labial margin or the appearance will be compromised.

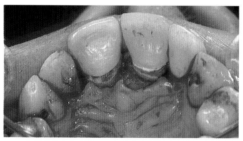

a

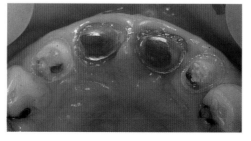

b

Figure 7.40 (a) Defective palatal crown margins with resulting caries. (b) Surgery was necessary to expose the margins but much dentine had been lost. Cast-gold post and cores were made with palatal diaphragms to restore the lost structure and prevent future fracture

Chapter 8

Restoration of posterior teeth

Treatment of teeth with extensive caries

While major loss of coronal dentine in an anterior tooth requiring a crown most frequently leads to a decision to make a post and core – after endodontic treatment if this has not already been carried out – the situation with posterior teeth is different. Here it is frequently possible to provide sufficient support and retention for a crown without resorting to endodontics and the provision of a post. In most instances it is possible to build up the general shape of the tooth by providing a core of amalgam, composite resin or glass ionomer cement. These cores are frequently retained by pins.

Pre-operative assessment

When confronted with a severely broken down tooth, the operator must first decide if the extent of tooth loss, due to caries, pre-existing restorations or other causes, is so severe that the tooth cannot be restored. With modern techniques this is rarely the case unless the tooth loss extends deeply subgingivally. As a general guide it may be considered that where more than half of the clinical crown is lost a core will be required to support and retain a crown or other cast restoration.

The pulpal status of the tooth must be assessed to determine if endodontic treatment will be required, or if this has already been completed, to determine if it is satisfactory.

The periodontal status and occlusal relationships of the tooth must, of course, also be considered.

Materials

Amalgam
In most instances amalgam is a very satisfactory core material. It is strong, can be used to restore smaller defects in retentively-shaped cavities and also major defects, with the aid of pins to provide retention for the material (Figures 8.1 and 8.2).

An amalgam core can effectively provide increased retention and resistance for a crown preparation, as well as minimizing the amount of metal required for a cast restoration. When a well-fitting copper band is used to support the amalgam the material can be built-up to retain the occlusal

Figure 8.1 (a) Caries removed from lower left molars. Pins and cement base placed. (b) Copper bands supporting condensed amalgam to maintain occlusal stability. (c) Completed crowns

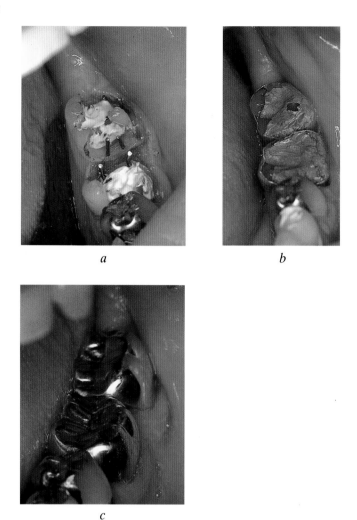

a

b

c

position until the crown is prepared. The only major disadvantage of the material is that it must be allowed to set until the next visit before crown preparation is undertaken. A further consideration is the darkening of the natural tooth that may be seen if a partial veneer crown is placed over an amalgam core. In this situation a composite core is generally to be preferred.

Composite resin
This material may be used as an alternative to amalgam in most situations. However, it is essential to maintain excellent moisture control and to build-up the core in increments, curing each fully before adding the next, in order to minimize the effects of polymerization contraction.

Composite resin has the particular advantage that in some situations its retention may be achieved by the use of a dentine bonding agent, and etching any residual enamel thereby reducing, or in some situations eliminating, the need for pins. Also, crown preparation may be done at the same visit that the core is placed and, with a partial veneer crown, the colour

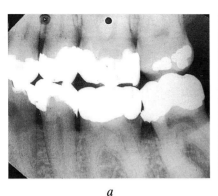
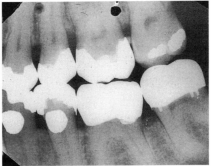

a   *b*

Figure 8.2 (a) Pre-operative radiographs showing defective restorations and caries. (b) Postoperative radiograph showing completed crowns

will probably be better than if an amalgam core had been used. It is not suitable, however, if the preparation extends subgingivally and the preparation must extend beyond the composite core. Composite is particularly useful in providing a core in conjunction with a pre-formed post (see Chapter 7).

Glass ionomer cement

This may be used if there is a considerable amount of crown remaining. It is adhesive to dentine and therefore pins are not normally needed, but it is not as strong as either amalgam or composite resins, so should not be used in stressed situations.

Cermet

Glass ionomers with the addition of metals are sometimes advocated as core materials. However, they appear to be less satisfactory than unmodified glass ionomer cements since their adhesion to dentine is less and mechanically they are no stronger.

Cast post and core

There is a considerable choice of materials and techniques available for posts and cores. Some of these are suitable for posterior as well as anterior teeth. They are discussed and described in Chapter 7.

Preparation sequence

All peripheral caries must first be removed, together with previous restorations, unless they are recent and have an approved history. Unsupported tooth tissue must also be removed unless it is to be retained as part of the core foundation.

Any central staining should be removed only if there is softening of the dentine. Isolated areas of stained dentine overlying the pulp are best dealt with by indirect pulp capping.

Retention may be improved by incorporating grooves or boxes in the preparation and by converting sloping surfaces into vertical and horizontal components.

Pin(s) or post(s) may be incorporated to increase retention, then a base inserted in the usual way and the core material built-up. The construction of a pin-retained amalgam core, which is the most generally satisfactory material, is described in detail.

Pin-retained amalgam

There are several types of pin used to provide additional retention for amalgam and any of these can be used in the construction of a pin-retained amalgam core.

The two main types are:

1. Friction retained pins, which require a slightly undersized pin-hole.
2. Threaded pins which cut their own thread into the dentine walls of a pre-drilled hole. These provide considerably more retention than the other types and have largely superseded type 1.

There are different varieties of threaded pins, but the safest and easiest to use has a bur shank that locks directly into a standard contra-angle handpiece. Thus the pin is held securely and there is little danger of it being inhaled or swallowed by the patient. These pins are made of stainless steel and come in two diameters with matching twist drills. The length of the thread is 4 mm.

1. Standard pins 0.76 mm diameter inserted into an 0.68 mm diameter pin-hole.
2. Thinner pins 0.60 mm diameter inserted into an 0.53 mm diameter pin-hole.

The depth of pin-hole is limited to approximately 2 mm by the shoulder of the twist drill and this allows the remaining 2 mm of thread to project from the dentine.

The pins can be bent once they are in position when it is necessary to ensure that they become completely embedded in the amalgam. A simple bending tool is readily made by cutting a notch in the blade of a discarded hand instrument.

Pins add considerably to the retention of amalgam in large cavities but they also weaken the amalgam. Thus only the number of pins that will provide the necessary additional retention should be used. As a rule of thumb, one pin for each missing cusp is a minimum requirement.

The pins must be sited in dentine but never so close together or to adjacent cavity walls as to prevent the proper condensation of amalgam around each pin (Figures 8.3 and 8.4).

Technique:

1. Make a starting pit in dentine approximately 1 mm from the enamel–dentine junction using a size half-round bur. This gives a positive location and prevents the twist drill slipping on the dentine surface.
2. Using the appropriate twist drill, prepare the pin-hole in dentine parallel with the adjacent external tooth surface. This reduces the risk of perforating into the pulp or periodontal ligament.

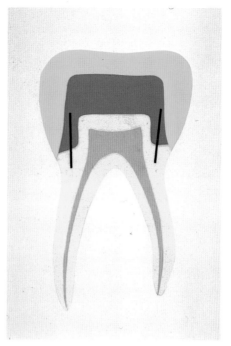

Figure 8.3 The position of pins is important. They should be within dentine, avoiding both pulp and cementum. This may require them to be inserted in a direction not in the long axis of the tooth. They should allow space for the amalgam to be condensed around them

3. Wash the pin-holes with a warm air–water spray but dry with paper points to avoid dehydration. The prepared holes may be protected with a lining of cavity varnish.
4. The pin should then be positioned and in the case of the threaded pin described, the shank is first latched into a contra-angle handpiece. The pin is screwed into the pre-drilled hole at a very slow speed and it will shear off at the neck when it has threaded into the 2 mm of pin-hole.
5. If necessary each pin is bent into the cavity so as to be within the confines of the proposed amalgam core.

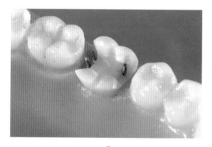

a

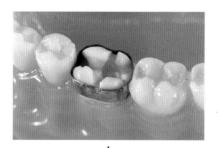

b

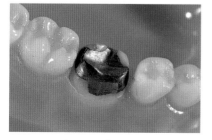

c

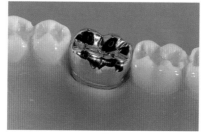

d

Figure 8.4 (a) Cavity prepared and pins inserted. (b) Copper band contoured gingivally and trimmed clear of the occlusion. (c) Pin-retained amalgam core. Note that the preparation extends beyond the amalgam. (d) Completed gold veneer crown

Figure 8.5 (a) Completed root filling in lower molar. (b) Radiograph showing amalgam condensed into the prepared pulp chamber and built up for the amalgam core. (c) The completed amalgam core is prepared for a full veneer crown

a

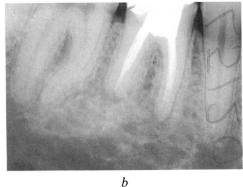

b

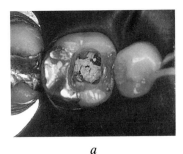

c

A copper band makes a convenient matrix for the amalgam, as it is thick, and when removed leaves the amalgam out of contact with the adjacent teeth. This allows easier preparation of the approximal surfaces. It is usual for the copper band to be left in place until the next visit, provided it has been trimmed to ensure that it does not interfere with the occlusion. The amalgam is thus given support and tooth movement is prevented.

At the next visit the tooth is prepared for a veneer crown, treating the amalgam as sound tooth substance. The outline of the veneer crown preparation should, however, extend onto sound tooth substance beyond the amalgam core by at least 1 mm.

It should be remembered that not all pulpless teeth necessarily require posts (Figure 8.5). Even cores are not required in all instances, but it is essential to ensure there is a sound base on which any crown or cast restoration is placed.

Full gold veneer crowns

Gold can be cast accurately in thin sections, which resist repeated stress without breaking or flexing. It is, therefore, ideal for use as a protective veneer. When this cover is extended over all the surfaces of a clinical crown it is called a full veneer crown. The thickness of a veneer can be varied as necessary to suit the functional demands of a remodelled occlusal surface or to recontour other surfaces of a tooth.

The gold veneer can be a single unit, form a strong junction with other units of a bridge or carry attachments for a removable denture.

Retention is obtained from opposing axial walls, which should be near parallel. However, when the clinical crown of a posterior tooth has lost much tooth tissue through caries or fracture, the best solution is to restore the lost tissue with an amalgam core, sometimes pin-retained. An existing amalgam restoration may be used as the core if it is sound and sufficiently retentive. This core can be shaped in the same manner as the tooth and it is then fully covered by the veneer.

The restoration of posterior teeth with extensive carious destruction or existing large amalgam restorations is simplified by the use of amalgam cores, which assist in the retention of the gold veneer crown.

Indications and contra-indications

1. When a full veneer cover is necessary, gold is the material of choice because it requires minimal tooth reduction.
2. A tooth weakened by endodontic treatment that involved much tissue loss intra-coronally is well protected by a gold veneer. This also applies to posterior teeth with intra-coronal buccal and lingual restorations.
3. Intra-coronal attachments or rest seats for partial dentures are easily incorporated in a full gold crown.
4. When appearance is not a significant factor, a full gold crown is often used as a bridge retainer. It offers good retention and requires minimal tooth reduction.
5. When constructing a full gold crown, the technician can incorporate undercuts for partial denture clasps or contour the buccal surface of the crown so that food is properly deflected.

There are no absolute contra-indications to full gold veneer crowns but the following points should be remembered:

1. Teeth with very short or tapering clinical crowns may require additional retention in the form of pins or slots.
2. A full gold veneer crown does not offer a good appearance and most patients would probably object to such a restoration in the anterior or middle region of the arch. It would therefore have to be restricted to the second or third molar regions.

Specific considerations

1. The health of the pulp. If this is in doubt appropriate endodontic treatment should be completed before proceeding further.
2. The extent of any caries. It is important to decide if the pulp may be in any danger of carious exposure and how far gingivally the caries has extended. The treatment of teeth with extensive caries is described on pages 99 to 104.
3. Existing restorations to be covered by the crown. Those which are suspect must be removed and the cavities dealt with as described in Chapter 1.
4. The potential of the remaining natural crown for retention. Short tapered clinical crowns with less than 4 mm vertical height will need some additional retention.

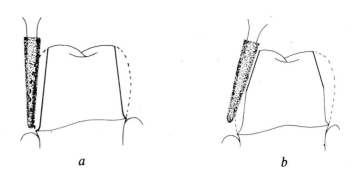

a   *b*

5. The crown margins. There is no reason why the margins of a gold crown cannot finish on an existing amalgam restoration provided that this has been thoroughly investigated and found to be sound, and that a minimum of 2 mm amalgam remains cervically to the crown margin.

Preparation for full gold veneer crowns

The preparation of a lower molar tooth for a full gold veneer crown is described and illustrated. Similar principles apply to the preparation of other posterior teeth.

1. Buccal and lingual surface reduction

A tapered diamond point (coarse grade) with a rounded end is used for the reduction of the buccal and lingual surfaces. It is important to have a clear idea of the path of withdrawal at this stage because this will largely determine the amount of tooth substance to be removed. The object is not to remove a layer of tooth as if peeling an onion but to establish a cervical collar that is as long as possible with walls that taper no more than 5° (Figure 8.6a). Sufficient tooth is removed to establish the axial walls and to define a cavo-surface angle immediately above the gingival margin. An untouched section of tooth may then still remain between the prepared axial wall and the occlusal surface, especially on an upper molar. This is then reduced sufficiently to allow for the correct contour of the finished crown (Figure 8.6b). Failure to remove enough tooth at this stage will result in a bulbous crown, but there is no need to remove all the enamel if all these conditions have been satisfied.

As a rule, the margins of a full gold veneer crown are placed supragingivally. However, this may be difficult or even impossible when dealing with a short clinical crown.

2. Approximal reduction

Approximal surfaces may be reduced using a fine tapered instrument. The type with a rounded tip is particularly convenient as it lessens the risk of damage to the gingival margins (Figure 8.7).

Reduction is continued until all undercut is removed approximally and the prepared surfaces extend to the gingival crest and converge a maximum of 5° towards the occlusal surface.

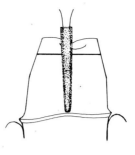

Figure 8.7 Preparation of the approximal surfaces to complete the cervical collar

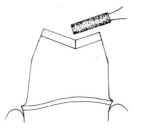

Figure 8.8 Preparation of the occlusal surface to allow sufficient clearance from opposing teeth

3. Occlusal surface reduction

The occlusal surface is reduced sufficiently to allow space for 1 mm of gold to cover it (Figure 8.8). A cylindrical diamond may be used for this reduction. The general shape of the prepared surface should be similar to that of the tooth itself, but it may be necessary to remove a greater amount of tissue in the fissures than elsewhere to ensure that all caries has been removed. Deepening the fissures also increases resistance of the crown to displacement. This should be done with a tapered fissure tungsten–carbide bur or diamond instrument.

After the occlusal surface has been reduced, it is important that the occlusion is checked in all positions of the mandible, to ensure that sufficient tissue has been removed. It is helpful to get the patient to close into 1 mm thick wax in intercuspal position to reveal areas of inadequate clearance.

A thicker occlusal section must be provided where teeth show heavy occlusal wear facets as these are evidence of damaging parafunctional movements causing extra stress and wear. A simple additional precaution is to persuade such patients to wear an acrylic splint, covering incisal and occlusal surfaces, at night if the nocturnal bruxism has not been eliminated.

4. Finishing the preparation

The junction of occlusal and axial surfaces should be rounded slightly, but excessive reduction will lead to some loss of retention. The axial walls should be re-checked at this stage and the gingival finishing line checked for definition (Figure 8.9). Clarity of this finishing line is essential to enable the technician to form a wax pattern with a clearly defined margin and thereby ensure a perfect marginal seal and a non-bulging contour of the completed crown.

Figure 8.9 Finished preparation showing rounded angles

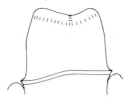

Diamond instruments that will produce an adequately finished cavo-surface angle of 135° should be used. Sharp angles between the occlusal and axial walls should be rounded lightly.

Except where conditions dictate otherwise the finishing line should be kept just supragingival in a position where the patient can clean the junction between tooth and crown.

Additional retention

In the section dealing with contra-indications it was mentioned that teeth with short or tapered clinical crowns may require further retention in addition to that obtained in the standard preparation. The usual ways of gaining this are:

1. The use of pins in the occlusal surface. Pin-holes may be prepared as for pin-retained inlays and iridio–platinum pins incorporated in the finished casting. The position of the pulp should always be assessed before the retention holes are cut.
2. The placing of grooves in the approximal surfaces, similar to those for partial gold veneer crowns. Grooves may also be placed in the buccal and lingual surfaces.

Impressions for full gold veneer crowns

The various indirect impression techniques suitable for veneer crowns are discussed in Chapter 5.

Temporary restorations

Temporary cover and protection of the prepared tooth is discussed in Chapter 4. However, teeth prepared for full gold veneers sometimes have very short clinical crowns, particularly after the completion of the preparation. In such situations the use of aluminium crown forms, which are available in various sizes, are helpful. They can be cut and adapted to the tooth prior to cementation with zinc oxide cement.

Fitting and cementing the crown

The procedure of trying-in, cementing and finishing a full gold veneer crown is similar to that of gold inlays or other types of veneer crowns.

Particular care should be taken to ensure that the crown is fully seated onto the prepared tooth. It is not always easy to determine if the crown has its margins entirely within the gingival sulcus. The curvature of the buccal and lingual walls must also be checked, because, in the interest of gingival health, the crown must reproduce the optimum contour of the tooth.

When cementing a full crown it is sometimes difficult to seat it completely as a result of trapped air or cement. The relief of the internal occlusal surface of the crown is a satisfactory way to overcome this problem. This relief may be provided by an appropriate die spacer on the occlusal and axial surfaces of the die in the laboratory stages.

Alternatively, a channel or groove may be cut with a round bur down the fitting surface of the crown from the occlusal surface to 1 mm from the margin.

Metal–ceramic crowns

The main reason for the frequent use of this crown is its versatility. It combines strength with an acceptable appearance and can be used either as a single unit or as a retainer in bridgework.

It is a full veneer metal crown with porcelain covering one or more of its surfaces. The preparation of the tooth has the palatal surface finished by a chamfer whereas the buccal or labial margins are finished similarly to a porcelain jacket crown. The shoulder is wide so that it can accommodate both the metal substructure and the porcelain. But it should have an acceptable appearance without the crown being overcontoured.

Views regarding the design of the crown often differ with regards to the junction between metal and porcelain. Some operators feel this should be on the palatal slope of the buccal cusp, therefore having porcelain covering the buccal surface and most of the buccal cusp or cusps. However, other operators feel it is the porcelain that makes this crown so much better in appearance than gold crowns. Therefore, whenever sufficient tissue can be removed from the occlusal surface of the tooth to be prepared there is no reason why the porcelain should not cover the whole of the occlusal, proximal and most of the palatal surfaces (Figure 8.10). At the palatal

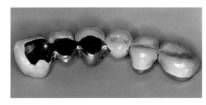

a

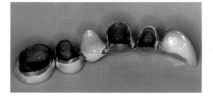

b

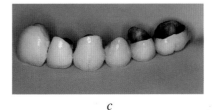

c

Figure 8.10 (a) A metal–ceramic bridge with full porcelain cover on both posterior retainers. Note the palatal shamfered margins where only metal forms the marginal edge of the retainers. (b) The same bridge showing the anterior labial retainer margins in porcelain. (c) The labial aspect of the bridge has proximal spaces with good access for cleaning devices. Interproximal staining of the porcelain can also be seen

Figure 8.11 (a) Butt joint shoulder margin design with metal collar finished just short of buccal preparation margin for optimum appearance. (b) Bevelled shoulder margin with metal collar cervically to give strength and optimal fit when the buccal margin is not visible or appearance is not critical. (c) Shamfer margin preparation design is preferred when a minimal preparation is required or the preparation has to be extended cervically onto the root

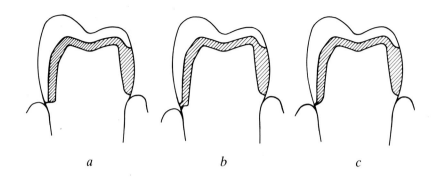

a   *b*   *c*

margin the last 1 mm continues to form the finishing chamfer in metal only. It is accepted that in some cases this might cause slight differential wear of the opposing tooth. Furthermore, full porcelain coverage of the occlusal surface requires more occlusal reduction of the preparation and this design is therefore not suitable for every case.

The junction between porcelain and metal should not be anywhere near an area where the opposing tooth makes contact. Contact in the area where half the occlusal force is on metal and the other half on porcelain, will cause damage resulting in a fracture of the porcelain.

There are various margin designs, and for the posterior metal ceramic crown the bevelled shoulder margins improve the marginal adaptation of the crown. The interproximal and palatal surfaces can be finished by a simple chamfer in order to minimize tooth reduction (Figure 8.11).

The metal substructure must be contoured to support the porcelain adequately to result in a near even thickness of porcelain cover. Overbuilt porcelain unsupported by metal may allow cohesive failure to occur within the material, resulting in porcelain fracture. This is an area where good communication between the dentist and the technician is essential to avoid a possible fracture of porcelain at some later date (Figure 8.12).

The preparation

The preparation of a posterior tooth for a metal ceramic crown differs little from that for a gold veneer crown. However, the following points must be stressed:

1. In order to accommodate the metal and porcelain buccally considerable reduction of the tooth is necessary on that surface. A reduction of

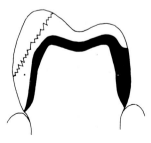

Figure 8.12 Overbuilt porcelain unsupported by metal may allow cohesive failure within the porcelain cover

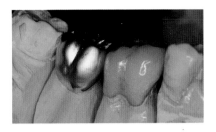

Figure 8.13 Two well-contoured molar crowns. The distal crown was grit-blasted to minimize the high gloss reflection of the gold. The metal–ceramic crown has a full porcelain cover. Note the concave contour near the bifurcation on both crowns

1.5 mm is the minimum required for an adequate thickness of porcelain, although this can be tapered off to 1 mm near the cervical shoulder preparation.
2. Occlusally, the preparation depends very much on the opposing teeth but inadequate reduction of this surface is a common fault, resulting in fracture of porcelain, which is too thin because of insufficient room. If there is an area of insufficient room for both metal and porcelain, then it is best to leave a metal 'island' without a porcelain cover rather than risk a porcelain fracture.
3. The interproximal and palatal or lingual surfaces are finished to a chamfer. When the porcelain is extended over the whole of the palatal surface it should terminate 1 mm short of the margin, which will be in metal only.

The impression techniques, finishing and cementing of the crown are described elsewhere. However, some points dealing with the appearance of the crown must be mentioned here.

Shade selection
Posterior teeth do not have just one shade. In particular the posterior teeth of older people have a variety of shades. It is therefore important to avoid the appearance of a unicoloured, near white blob in the arch.

1. Cervical staining is common in older people and a crown should also include this darker staining.
2. Interproximal surfaces sometimes have a slightly orange appearance and if so this should be reproduced on the crown.
3. Occlusally, natural teeth often have fissure staining. Crowns should be no different. When adjacent teeth have fissure staining this should be copied on the crown.

Gold inlays and onlays

Gold inlays were prepared originally by a technique similar to that used for porcelain inlays. A gold or platinum foil matrix was adapted to the cavity and then carefully removed and filled to the correct contour with gold solder. Taggart in 1907 adapted the lost-wax technique of the 'ancients' and produced cast-gold inlays. Today a variety of casting alloys has been developed and an alloy can be selected to suit the demands of a particular restoration. Modern inlay waxes and investment techniques make dimensional control possible so that a casting in the alloy may have an accuracy within the limits of $\pm 0.2\%$, and for an average inlay casting this represents $\pm 10\,\mu$m. The importance of precision in all inlay work must be emphasized because a bad inlay is a hazard to the tooth and a disservice to the patient.

The advantages of the inlay over its rival, amalgam, are mainly due to the strength of the alloy from which the inlay is constructed. The strength is important to resist distortion under masticatory load and because thin sections or veneers of gold may be used to protect weak parts of the tooth. An intracoronal gold inlay relies on the strength of the remaining tooth structure for its support and retention. Sufficient bulk of tooth substance is needed to resist any wedging effect on the preparation walls. The inlay merely replaces missing tooth structure and does not reinforce the tooth. This restoration is contra-indicated in a significantly weakened tooth. Three surface (MOD) inlays should be restricted to situations in which the isthmus can be kept narrow (¼ to ⅓ the intercuspal width). Otherwise the occlusal surface of the tooth should be reduced to convert the preparation into a gold onlay. This occlusal coverage with an extracoronal veneer of casting alloy redistributes occlusal forces over a wide area and protects the remaining tooth tissue from fracture.

There are a number of situations in which inlays are generally contra-indicated. They are not, for instance, satisfactory in very small, shallow cavities. Some patients object to their appearance in anterior teeth, although a facing may disguise an obvious display of gold. It is wiser not to attempt inlay restorations on patients whose oral hygiene is poor and whose dentition has been neglected. Similarly, they are contra-indicated for patients with rampant caries because of the frequent need to extend restorations as a result of caries recurring at their margins.

Cavity preparation

For inlay work the dual objectives in cavity preparation are to remove the caries and shape the cavity for an effective restoration.

Caries

The final outline of the cavity depends on the extent of the carious lesion. Where it is minimal, an initial penetration is made just into the dentine and the cavity is extended at this optimal depth to the classic outline. This outline is determined by the class of cavity, the tooth form and the need to remove adjacent stagnation areas on the tooth surface. At no point should the margin of the cavity cross a caries-susceptible area, such as a fissure. A small carious lesion is often completely removed when establishing a classic outline at the optimal depth. If not, the lesion is at least isolated, leaving only a small area of caries on the pulpal floor to be excavated.

A larger carious lesion will have caused some breakdown of the enamel surface with obvious cavitation. Here the first stage is to remove undermined enamel in order to obtain access to the lesion. Carious dentine at the enamel–dentine junction is then removed until the periphery is sound. Undermined enamel is next removed and any remaining fissures are included within the cavity outline. At this stage the outline of the cavity is only decided provisionally because subsequent modification may become necessary following the alignment of internal walls to the path of withdrawal or the reduction of weakened cusps. Caries remaining in the centre of the cavity has to be dealt with in the usual way. If the lesion is deep the integrity of the pulp must be considered before proceeding further.

Resistance and retention

It is axiomatic that an inlay must withstand the forces exerted on it and that it must stay in the cavity. Resistance to occlusal stress is generally obtained by providing flat pulpal and gingival floors for the cavity, if necessary by the addition of a cement base over the pulp. Resistance to lateral stress is provided by an occlusal lock and by axial walls. For good retention an inlay must have a single path of insertion into its cavity, in a direction that is usually in line with the main occlusal load; masticatory forces will then tend to seat the inlay more securely into its cavity. This single path of insertion is achieved by near parallelism of the cavity walls so that the inlay can be displaced only along the path of its insertion. The friction provided between the near parallel walls and the inlay when it is cemented will prevent this displacement.

Cavo-surface angles

The marginal integrity of an inlay depends on the existence of well-defined cavo-surface angles. These are usually cut in enamel, and if left unfinished or only crudely finished, they are a potential hazard to the life of an inlay. Crumbling of a margin due to minor irregularities, not necessarily visible to the naked eye, can lead to recurrence of caries. Therefore, these margins must be smoothed and finished with great care. In addition, a cavo-surface angle must be designed to allow burnishing of the gold margins to the tooth.

In practice the minimum cavo-surface angle that permits a thin enough cover of gold capable of being burnished is about 135°. This special preparation of the margin of an inlay cavity is referred to as 'bevelling'. Bevels usually extend through half the thickness of enamel except cervically, where the enamel is thinner, and here the full thickness of enamel is bevelled (Figures 8.14 to 8.17). The method of obtaining the correct cavo-surface angle in each situation is described with the appropriate cavity.

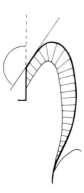

Figure 8.14 The cavo-surface angle is greater than 135°. Bevel is not required

Figure 8.15 The cavo-surface angle in (a) is bevelled to produce an angle of 135° as shown in (b)

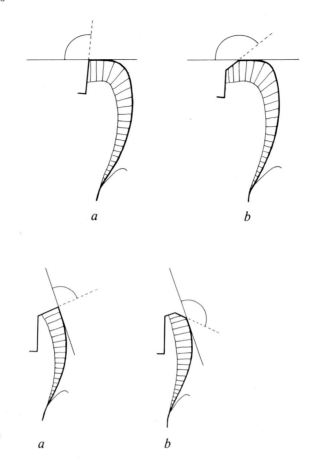

a   *b*

Figure 8.16 The cavo-surface angle in (a) is bevelled to produce an angle of 135° as shown in (b)

a   *b*

Figure 8.17 Cervically the full thickness of the enamel is bevelled to produce an angle of 135°

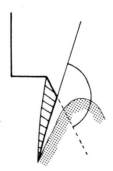

Cavity lining

When the cavity is caries-free, clean and dry, it should be lined with a cement base where necessary. This enables any minor undercuts in the dentine to be lined out and provides a flat floor to the cavity. It also avoids the use of unnecessarily large amounts of gold. Very deep parts of a cavity should have a sub-base of calcium hydroxide to protect the pulp.

A cement base cannot add to retention or resistance but a poor one may seriously detract from a good preparation. It is very easy to make a cavity too shallow with a base or in other ways to spoil good preparations by obliterating detail.

Temporary dressings

Cast restorations cannot be fitted immediately after cavity preparation and, therefore, a temporary restoration will have to be placed in the cavity until the inlay is ready.

Zinc oxide and eugenol types of cement must be used as a temporary dressing where there are freshly-cut dentinal tubules; a quick-setting variety makes a satisfactory temporary restoration for inlay work. The incorporation of cotton-wool fibres to toughen the cement and a thin coating of petroleum jelly facilitates its removal. Where cusps have been reduced, a resin onlay should be made using an impression of the unprepared tooth (see Chapter 4 for technique).

Wherever pins are used, the pin-holes must not be obliterated with temporary dressing and to prevent this a cotton-wool plug or a paper point is inserted into each pin-hole. Pre-formed pins in steel or plastic may also be used.

The class II cavity

The approximal occlusal restoration, MO, DO, or MOD, is by far the most common in conservative dentistry. The basic principles governing the preparation of cavities for inlays has already been dealt with, but it is worth restating that the finished cavity for an inlay must have a single path of insertion and opposing near parallel walls that form sharp internal angles with a flat floor. The cavity must also resist displacement of the inlay by lateral stresses. As well as an occlusal box the Class II cavity has an approximal part with buccal and lingual walls and these have to be extended so that the margins are just accessible for cleaning by the patient. The enamel walls also have to be finished with a cavo-surface angle of at least 135°. These aims can be achieved with a box preparation.

The MO or DO box preparation
The shape of the cavity, when there is minimal caries, is shown in Figure 8.18. This preparation consists of an occlusal part in dovetail form and an

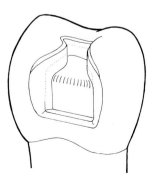

Figure 8.18 Class II box cavity

approximal box. The stages in the preparation of such a minimal cavity in an upper premolar will be described.

1. Access. A small tungsten–carbide bur at ultra-speed is used to cut just within the marginal ridge, and to penetrate along the enamel–dentine junction to the approximal caries.

2. Extension of approximal box. The proximal cut is extended to gingival level with a fine, tapered fissure bur at ultra-speed. The occlusogingival depth can be measured on the side of the tooth for guidance (Figure 8.19a). While establishing the gingival floor, sweeping cuts are made buccally and lingually to outline the lateral extent of the approximal box. The enamel which is undermined by this procedure (Figure 8.19a, b) is removed with a chisel or hatchet (Figure 8.20). It is important to retain the enamel until this stage so that the adjacent tooth is protected from the bur. The tapered fissure bur at ultra-speed is then used to remove any irregularities of the approximal box and to flatten the gingival floor. At the same time angles are cut where the floor meets the buccal wall on one side, the lingual wall on the other, and the axial wall which joins them (Figure 8.21).

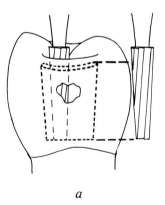
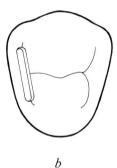

Figure 8.19 (a) Approximal box formation within the approximal enamel. (b) Primary extension of the approximal box

a

b

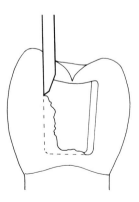

Figure 8.20 Removing undermined approximal enamel

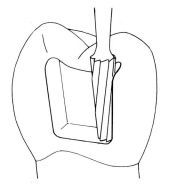

Figure 8.21 Flattening the gingival floor and sharpening the angles it makes with other walls

3. Outline of occlusal form. A tapered fissure bur at ultra-speed is used to outline the occlusal part of the preparation. The cut should be just into dentine and extended for various teeth as indicated (Figures 8.22 to 8.25). The occlusal outline is virtually identical to the outline of a Class I cavity preparation and it is really immaterial whether this or the approximal box is cut first. The preparation margin should end at least 1 mm away from the nearest occlusal contact.

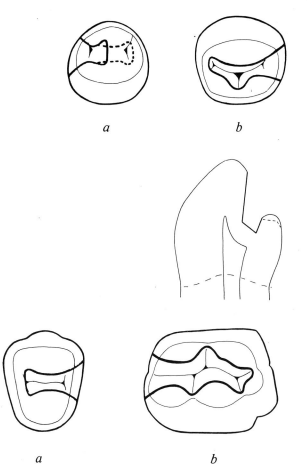

a

b

Figure 8.22 (a) Alternative outlines for the occlusal dovetail in the lower first premolar. (b) Outline for the occlusal dovetail in a lower second premolar

Figure 8.23 Pulpal floor angle in a lower premolar, which avoids undermining the lingual cusp and exposing the pulp. Frequently, the lingual cusp is weak and requires protection

a

b

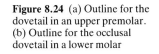

Figure 8.24 (a) Outline for the dovetail in an upper premolar. (b) Outline for the occlusal dovetail in a lower molar

Figure 8.25 (a) Alternative
outlines for the occlusal dovetail
of a mesial cavity in an upper
molar. (b) Alternative outlines for
the occlusal dovetail of a distal
cavity in an upper molar

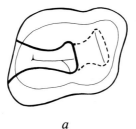 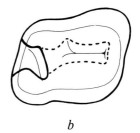

a   *b*

4. Finishing the approximal box. The approximal box is completed using an enamel chisel to plane its vertical walls and to sharpen the line angles. The enamel margins are finished. It may be necessary, at this stage, to flare the buccal and lingual enamel walls with a flame-shaped diamond, in order to achieve the optimum cavo-surface angle (Figure 8.26). The gingival enamel is finished with a bladeless tungsten–carbide finisher or a flame-shaped carbide finishing bur. The carbide finishing bur is used to blend the gingival bevel with the buccal and lingual flares and to go over the flares to produce a smooth, well-defined, finish line.

5. Gingival lock. Although not essential to the cavity, it is possible to cut a groove with a reverse gingival margin trimmer into the dentine of the gingival floor. This will act as a lock under stress so that the inlay tends to seat more securely in the cavity (Figure 8.27).

6. Finishing the occlusal dovetail. The cut enamel surface of the occlusal dovetail is smoothed with a plain-cut bur and the cavo-surface angle is bevelled where necessary.

7. Caries removal and lining. Any caries remaining at the pulpal floor or axial wall is excavated and the defect is filled with cement (Figure 8.28). Deep excavations will need a protective sub-base.

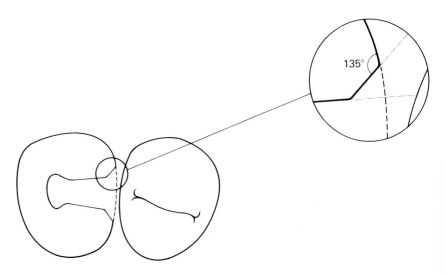

Figure 8.26 The flare of the cut
enamel walls

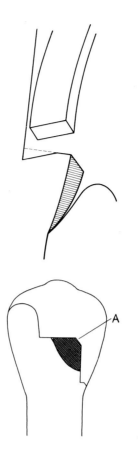

Figure 8.27 A lock made in the gingival floor of a cavity with a reversed gingival margin trimmer

-A

Figure 8.28 Cement (A) restoring localized excavation of carious dentine in a class II cavity

When free of debris and absolutely clean, the preparation is ready for the impression. The choice of material and technique for impressions are discussed in Chapter 5.

The extensive MO or DO cavity
When the approximal marginal ridge has already broken away or is seriously undermined by caries, the approach is different and stages 1–3, outlined for the preparation in the case of a minimal lesion, are different.

1. Access. The undermined enamel or marginal ridge is removed using a chisel.

2. Initial extension. The approximal and occlusal parts are extended to the limits suggested for the minimal cavity.

3. Removal of caries and final extension. The enamel–dentine junction of the cavity is excavated until it is clean and caries-free. All undermined enamel is then planed away until the enamel is based on sound dentine. This may result in the cavity being more extensive buccolingually than is necessary for a self-cleansing margin, but this is no problem for satisfactory restoration with an inlay, because inlay techniques permit excellent reconstruction of contour. However, any undercuts in the dentine that result from the removal of caries will have to be filled with a cement base.

Final stages. These are the same as stages 4–7 described for a minimal preparation.

It is important that before an MO or DO preparation is considered complete, reassessment should be made of the caries incidence and the chance of a new cavity developing on the unaffected approximal surface. An adequate occlusal dovetail is sometimes difficult to achieve in a large MO or DO cavity. To provide the necessary resistance, and also additional retention, the cavity should be extended into an MOD preparation. Alternatively, one or more pins may be incorporated into the inlay design to gain additional retention.

The MOD cavity

This cavity, with its combined mesial and distal parts, is more difficult to prepare because of the extra surfaces that must be kept to a common line of withdrawal.

Cusp coverage
Very often when the more extensive cavity has been excavated free of caries and extended 'for prevention' one or more cusps are left weak. If these weakened cusps remain unprotected there is a danger that they will fracture during mastication. As a guide it can be assumed that if the cusp is higher than its base is broad then the protection of the cusp with gold is necessary (Figure 8.29). To obtain space for this layer of gold, the height of the cusp must be reduced. When all unsupported enamel has been removed the cusp reduction is made with a diamond instrument, at ultra-speed, until there is cuspal clearance of at least 1 mm in all excursions of the mandible. An extra 0.5 mm reduction may be indicated for functional cusps (palatal and mandibular buccal cusps). Adequacy of occlusal reduction should be assessed by direct visual inspection and where this is not possible (lingual cusps) utility wax may be used to assess reduction.

The buccal or lingual margin of reduced cusps should be bevelled to give a

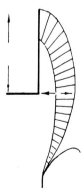

Figure 8.29 A cusp that is higher than its base is broad requires protection

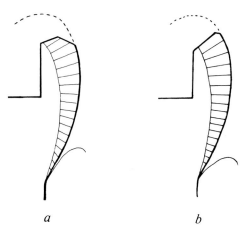

Figure 8.30 (a) A reverse bevel is used to finish the buccal margin of a reduced lower cusp. (b) A reverse bevel on a buccal margin of an upper tooth

a   *b*

cavo-surface angle of about 135° and this is referred to as a reverse bevel (Figure 8.30). The margin of the bevel should be extended to ensure that the full movement of opposing cusps is on the restoration and does not cross from enamel to gold, otherwise the margin of the restoration would soon be damaged. Therefore, it is necessary to extend the cover more on the buccal cusp of a lower tooth than on an upper tooth. (The reverse is the situation for palatal/lingual functional cusp bevels.)

It is in these circumstances of weakened tooth substance that the strength of gold casting alloys become so important. Partial or complete coverage of an occlusal surface will give protection to vulnerable tissue and prevent its fracture. This is often necessary when large amalgam restorations have failed and are being replaced. In addition, when enamel appears to be cracked or crazed in a tooth being restored, that aspect of the tooth should be protected with occlusal coverage. Similarly root-filled teeth should be protected because the coronal dentine has usually been considerably thinned, and therefore the crown weakened, during endodontic treatment.

When all the caries has been removed from an MOD preparation there is sometimes a considerable amount of undercut tooth tissue with weakened cusps. Although the unsupported enamel must be planed away it is not always necessary to remove all undercuts within the dentine. These may be lined out with cement after a suitable sub-base has been inserted (Figure 8.31).

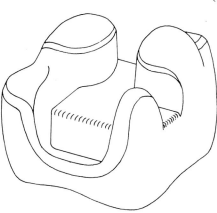

Figure 8.31 Complex MOD molar cavity with weakened cusps reduced and a buccal groove extension

Additional retention is often necessary when caries has destroyed tissue that should have formed one of the axial walls of the cavity. In this situation one or more pins sunk into the floor of the cavity can make an important contribution to the retention and stability of the inlay. Matching dental twist drills, headed plastic impression pins, iridio–platinum casting pins and aluminium pins for use with temporary restorations are available for this purpose. Pin-holes must be cut in sound dentine, clear of the enamel–dentine junction and in a position where there is least danger of entering the pulp or periodontal ligament. Any doubt should be resolved by viewing the pre-operative bitewing radiograph.

Trying-in and finishing inlays

Immediately before try-in the temporary dressing is removed. The cavity and inlay are cleaned free of debris and then washed and dried. The airway should be protected with a butterfly sponge pack. The following stages comprise the 'try-in':

1. The inlay is seated in the cavity and the whole of the margin explored carefully with a sharp probe for any deficiencies or ledges. Ideally, the transition from tooth to inlay should be imperceptible to a probe. If the inlay cannot be seated in the cavity the cause must be looked for, in the following sequence:
   a. There may be debris in the cavity or on the fitting surface of the inlay, or gingivae may have encroached into the cavity. The remedy is obvious; debris is removed and tags of gum are trimmed away.
   b. The approximal contour may be overbuilt. This fault is easily detected because dental floss cannot be passed between the inlay and the adjacent tooth. The remedy is to disc away some of the gold from the contact area until the floss will just pass through the tight contact.
   c. The casting margin may have been over extended and the restoration may fail to seat fully until the over extension is removed.
   d. The impression may have been distorted. In this case it must be retaken, but before doing so the cavity should be re-examined to make certain that no undercut or roughness of its walls is responsible for the distortion. Attempts to modify a badly-fitting inlay are invariably fruitless so when the cause of the distorted impression has been identified and rectified, a new impression is taken.
2. If the inlay is acceptable as having a good marginal fit, the next step is to check with dental floss if contact with the adjacent tooth is firm enough. Small deficiencies of contact can be corrected with gold solder.
3. The occlusion must be checked in all excursions of the mandible and, where necessary, corrections made by spot grinding the inlay.

Cementing of gold inlays and onlays

Fine-grain cement is best for cementing dental restorations. This must be mixed to a smooth, creamy consistency that will not impede seating the inlay.

While the cavity is being dried and the field isolated with cotton-wool rolls, the casting is placed in 70% alcohol to facilitate drying. The cavity is finally inspected to make sure it is quite clean and dry. The inlay is dried and its fitting surface coated with the cement mix. The cavity may also be coated with the cement. The inlay is then seated firmly in position. A quick check of the occlusion will usually confirm that the casting has gone accurately into place. Pressure must be exerted on the restoration until the cement is set.

When the cement has set hard, the excess is fractured away from the margins with scalers or excavators. Particular care must be taken to remove excess cement from the gingival margins of the inlay because cement left in a gingival crevice will collect plaque and irritate the gingivae. Dental floss may be used to remove excess cement from interproximal areas.

Tooth-coloured inlays and onlays

Increasing aesthetic demands have led to more frequent use of tooth-coloured restorative materials in posterior teeth. Many patients are no longer willing to accept extensive gold inlays or onlays. Over the last decade a number of manufacturers have marketed composite and porcelain inlay systems for use in the posterior region of the mouth. These may offer a viable aesthetic alternative to the traditional gold inlay, especially in the premolar region of the mouth. They may be considered for patients who are regular dental attenders, who maintain a good standard of dental health and request the provision of tooth-coloured restorations.

Tooth-coloured restorations are suitable for teeth in which moderate to large-sized restorations are required, sufficient enamel remains for bonding and where the provision of a resin-bonded restoration is indicated to strengthen and protect the remaining tooth tissue. They offer an alternative to crowning as an intermediate to long-term restoration for endodontically treated teeth. In this situation the tooth may be too weak for amalgam, a cast-gold restoration may be unsuitable and a crown preparation too radical.

Resin-bonded inlays are contra-indicated where there is evidence of excessive tooth wear in relation to the patient's age, or there are signs and symptoms of bruxing, clenching or other chewing habits. A porcelain restoration may cause excessive wear of the opposing tooth/restoration and a composite inlay/onlay may have inadequate long-term wear resistance. They are also contra-indicated where there is inadequate tooth substance remaining to allow sufficient resistance and retention form to be created.

General considerations

Composite resin inlays may be classified according to the type of composite, method of curing and construction. Modern systems are manufactured from either microfilled composite (SR-Isosit: Vivadent) or fine particle hybrid composite (Brilliant: Coltene). They are cured using heat and pressure, heat and light or merely light. They are constructed by direct or indirect techniques. The latter includes both chairside and laboratory made inlays. Whilst laboratory made inlays require two appointments and the provision of a temporary restoration, they offer the best opportunity for producing a restoration of ideal contour and finish. Composite inlays should only be placed where the demands in terms of wear resistance and occlusal function are limited and where patients are prepared to accept restorations of unknown life-expectancy.

Ceramic restorations include castable materials (Dicor: Dentsply), materials fired on investment material (Flexo-Ceram Inlay System: Elephant Ceramics), and computer-aided ground materials (Cerec System: Siemens). When compared with composite inlays they have certain advantages including superior inertness, biocompatability and wear resistance in clinical service, and are generally preferred for onlay restorations. However, composite inlays are easier for the laboratory to make, less liable to fracture during try-in and cementation, and are easier to adjust, modify and refinish at the chairside. They are also easier to repair than ceramic inlays in the event of a failure.

Tooth preparation

The following characteristics describe the differences between gold and composite/porcelain inlay cavity preparations:

1. The taper for tooth-coloured inlay preparations should be increased compared to the 3 to 5° recommended for gold inlays. The materials used for these restorations are weak before cementation, and removing a near parallel inlay from the die or tooth preparation may be difficult and fracture can occur. A taper of 6 to 8° is recommended. Internal line and point angles are rounded.
2. Cavo-surface butt joint margins are recommended for occlusal and cervical cavity margins. In general, sharp margins and bevels create thin sections of brittle porcelain.
3. All cavity margins must be in enamel for optimal bonding and margins should also be supragingival to allow adequate moisture control during cementation. The final decision of whether a resin-bonded restoration is justified can only be made during the preparation itself.
4. Buccal and lingual box walls may be flared or bevelled to provide a greater surface area of enamel for etching and bonding.
5. Onlay preparations may have bevels placed on non-stress bearing buccal and lingual surfaces to provide better appearance by blending colours (Figure 8.32).

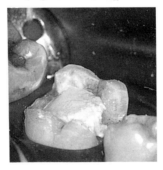
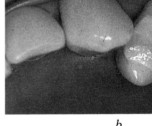

Figure 8.32 (a) Preparation for an MOD porcelain inlay with cuspal coverage. (b) The porcelain inlay of the upper first premolar has full buccal cusp coverage

a   *b*

6. All exposed dentine cavity surfaces are covered with a glass-ionomer lining at least 0.5 mm thick (Figure 8.33b). Internal undercuts are blocked out with glass-ionomer cement. If a light-cured material is used, this can be done at the same visit that the preparation is completed.
7. The occlusal isthmus width of an MOD cavity should be at least 2 mm and in a premolar cavity the occlusal isthmus width may typically be one third of the buccolingual width of the tooth. Because the cuspal support

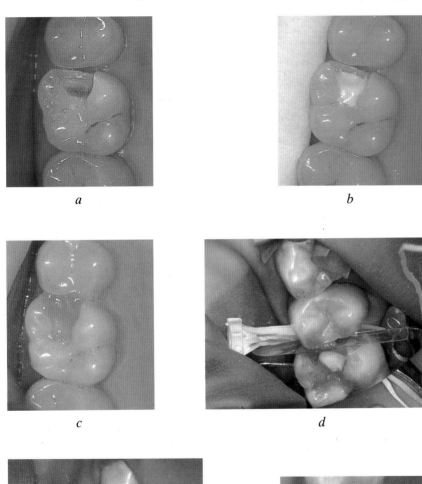

a

b

c

d

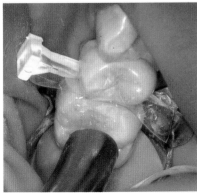

e

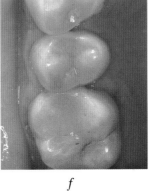

f

Figure 8.33 A sequence showing the use of a composite inlay in an upper molar tooth. (a) The prepared cavity. (b) The cavity is lined with glass-ionomer cement. (c) The temporary inlay (Fermit). (d) Rubber dam isolation. A clear matrix and light transmitting wedge. The etching gel is applied to the enamel margins. (e) Composite cement is cured with blue light. (f) The completed inlay

Figure 8.34 (a) The mesio-buccal cusp of |7 has fractured supra-gingivally. Sufficient enamel remains for acid-etch retention of a resin-bonded inlay. (b) Resin-bonded inlays in |567. Note the staining of fissures for characterization purposes

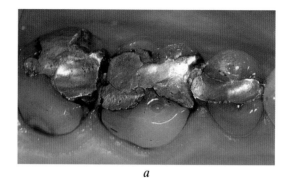

a

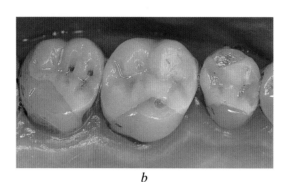

b

of a bonded restoration approaches that of a sound tooth there is less need for cuspal coverage than for a traditional gold restoration.
8. Cuspal reduction and extension is necessary when a cusp has fractured or is hopelessly undermined (Figure 8.34a, b). Cusp capping may also be required when the margin of an inlay approaches within 1 mm of an occlusal contact on a functional cusp that must withstand heavy occlusal loading. An occlusal clearance of 1.5 to 2.0 mm is required to allow for adequate material bulk.

Impression and temporary restoration

The impression technique is the same as for gold inlays. In the case of a simple inlay cavity the temporary restoration may be made using a soft, light-curing resin material (Fermit: Vivadent), which is placed in the cavity before asking the patient to occlude and grind on the uncured material. Excess material is removed, the patient is asked to occlude again and then the material is light cured for 60 sec. Larger inlay cavities and onlay preparations are best restored by an indirect technique using a chemically activated composite (Protemp II: Espe), which is cemented temporarily with a eugenol-free luting cement. Either a calcium hydroxide liner or a special eugenol-free temporary cement may be used for this purpose. It is important to trim the sectional silicone impression to the point where the impression is securely supported on the occlusal surfaces of the adjacent teeth so that occlusal adjustment of the temporary may be avoided. The cavity should be wetted before the resin is placed to facilitate removal of the cured material.

Shade selection and laboratory prescription

It is usually best to delay shade selection until cavity preparation is complete as old amalgam restorations may have altered the true colour of the tooth. Tooth-coloured inlays and onlays tend to blend in with the tooth colour very well even if there is a slight shade mismatch. Only the incisal one-third of the shade guide is required for assessment as most of these restorations will not involve the neck of the tooth. The laboratory prescription should include details such as the amount of any stain to be applied to any pits and fissures (Figure 8.34b).

Try-in and cementation

Because of their relatively weak and brittle nature, both try-in and cementation for ceramic and composite resin inlays and onlays are more demanding and time-consuming than for gold inlays.

The temporary restoration is removed and the preparation is cleaned with a slurry of pumice and water on a bristle brush to remove all debris and to clean the enamel cavity walls. A rubber dam is placed to ensure a dry field for acid-etching and bonding. The inlay is tried-in to verify internal and marginal fit and proximal contacts. Occlusal adjustment of porcelain inlays is best left until after cementation to avoid the possibility of fracture. The absence of an examination of the occlusion before bonding and the fragile nature of small porcelain inlays demands the highest possible precision from the dental technician. Near-perfect fit and function of the inlay/onlay on the mounted master cast is necessary as adjustment of the fit of the restoration in the mouth is very difficult.

When shade selection is critical to the success of the restoration it is best to delay rubber dam placement until the correct shade of resin cement has been decided. Nearly all inlays can be cemented successfully with a 'universal' shade of cement or one matching the shade of the restoration. During try-in, the inlay should not be forced into place. Minor marginal discrepancies may be acceptable as they will be filled with resin cement when bonding the restoration. The marginal fit may not equal that of a gold inlay but it should be very close and gross deficiencies cannot be accepted. The use of a silicone fit checker (Fit Checker: G. C. Dental) may contaminate the etched fit surface of a porcelain inlay/onlay and so the etched porcelain surface should be wetted beforehand if it is to be used. Dual-cured (light and chemically activated) composite resin luting cements are preferred for cementation of composite and porcelain inlays and onlays in order to enhance poly-merization of the luting composite in areas distant from the light source.

After try-in the inlay fit surface is cleaned with phosphoric acid applied for 15 sec. The acid is then rinsed off over a sink, which is partially filled with water to avoid possible loss or damage to the restoration. As these restorations are small and difficult to handle when wearing gloves, a handle attached to the occlusal surface of the restoration with sticky wax can be

Figure 8.35 Care is taken to ensure that the etching gel is only applied to the enamel margins

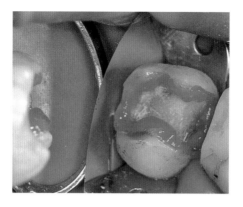

used. A silane bond enhancer is applied to the fit surface of the air-dried restoration if it is a ceramic or a hybrid composite resin inlay. A resin adhesion promoter (Special Bond II: Vivadent) should be applied to the fit surface of microfilled composite inlays immediately before cementation. The enamel cavity walls and margins of the preparation are acid-etched taking care to keep the etchant off adjacent teeth (Figure 8.35).

The glass-ionomer cement lining need not be etched. It is often necessary to isolate the tooth with matrix bands or strips during etching. It is also helpful to trim a clear contoured matrix band so that it covers the interproximal box area extending 1 mm gingival and 2 mm coronal to the box margin. It should then be trimmed apical to the contact area and it can be stabilized with a clear plastic wedge if necessary (Figure 8.33d). After etching, rinsing and drying, the mixed dual-cured unfilled resin adhesive is applied to the preparation and blown thin. Mixed dual-cure composite resin cement is applied to the fit surface of the restoration and it is seated gently into place. Gross excess cement is removed from the margins while holding the inlay in place with a blunt-ended instrument. A small amount of excess cement is left at the cavity margins.

The restoration is then 'tacked' into place by spot curing on the occlusal surface for 10 sec. Further excess cement is removed and the contacts are flossed, taking care not to move the restoration or cause bleeding by moving the floss too far gingivally. The use of a gingival matrix simplifies the finishing of this critical area. Once the cement begins its chemical cure and becomes 'doughy' no more excess should be removed as there is a risk of creating marginal voids. The inlay margins are covered with glycerine (Airblock: Dentsply) before light-curing to avoid the formation of an oxygen inhibited surface layer of luting composite, which greatly reduces wear resistance of the luting composite. Curing of the restoration is completed by directing light onto each buccal and lingual margin occlusally and interproximally for a minimum of 60 sec. per area.

After removal of the gingival matrix any excess cement remaining in this area may be removed with a number 12 scalpel blade or a tungsten–carbide tipped composite carver. Excess cement on the occlusal, buccal and lingual surfaces can be removed with composite finishing strips and diamonds. The gingival margin is smoothed, if necessary with aluminium oxide finishing

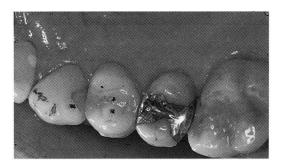

Figure 8.36 Occusal contacts in intercuspal position on 4| MOD ceramic inlay. Existence of a canine-guided occlusion reduces the possibility of excess wear of the opposing tooth

strips. The occlusion is checked and adjusted if necessary with finishing diamonds (Figure 8.36).

Final finishing is achieved with impregnated polishing points or 30-fluted finishing burs followed by a porcelain or composite polishing paste applied on a rubber cup. This may be carried interproximally with a finishing strip or dental tape. A final examination with an explorer on accessible surfaces and with dental floss interproximally is essential to exclude any composite resin overhangs. The patient is recalled one week later to reassess the occlusion and marginal adaptation.

Partial veneer crowns

The advantage of retaining the appearance and contours of a sound buccal or labial wall of a tooth is self-evident. The partial veneer crown makes this possible and was the most favoured bridge retainer before the advent of metal ceramic crowns. Retention is mainly gained by near parallelism of the approximal surfaces and deep slots placed into the approximal surfaces. The term 'three quarter crown' is frequently used for this restoration.

Indications and contra-indications

Even with a well designed partial veneer crown, the gold may still affect the colour of the restored tooth by altering its translucency. Therefore, this restoration is usually restricted to the posterior regions of the mouth. With the advent of metal ceramic materials, the gold partial veneer crown is only occasionally used in the anterior region of the mouth and then usually as the anterior retainer of a bridge.

It is not unusual for posterior teeth to have suffered severe lingual or palatal destruction, leaving the buccal wall virtually unaffected. The restoration of the missing tooth substance by a pin retained amalgam core and its subsequent protection by a partial veneer crown provides a satisfactory restoration. In such a case the amalgam–tooth junction should always be covered by gold.

The need for adequate retention between the two approximal slots and the lingual or palatal wall indicates that short clinical crowns or tapered clinical crowns are best avoided for partial veneer crowns.

These crowns are often used as retainers for short-span all-gold bridges.

However, because of the need for a reverse bevel on the occlusobuccal surface, gold will be visible. Therefore, this retainer is not always suitable in the premolar region of patients who do not like the appearance of gold in the mouth.

Clinical assessment of the tooth

A partial veneer crown has a longer periphery than a full veneer and should therefore only be considered when caries is not extensive and the patient's caries rate is low. The position of the pulp should always be assessed on radiographs to ensure that it is not damaged by the preparation of the retention grooves. This is particularly important if the tooth is to be a bridge abutment since the path of insertion of the crown will be determined by the other components of the bridge. The clinical length of the tooth and its bulk must be adequate for the retentive preparation and the support of a crown.

Preparation of posterior teeth for partial veneer crowns

1. Palatal reduction. The palatal surface is reduced with a tapered diamond instrument. The reduction is carried just to the gingival margin and must leave a surface that is nearly parallel to the planned line of withdrawal (Figure 8.37). The removal of undercuts is the main objective of this stage, and it is not always necessary to remove all the palatal enamel. Towards the occlusal surface, the contour of the tooth should be followed to provide an even thickness of gold. The best cervical fit will be obtained with a cavo-surface angle of 135° on a chamfer finishing line.

2. Approximal reduction. A fine tapered diamond instrument with a rounded tip is used at ultra-speed to prepare the approximal surfaces (Figure 8.38). They should be designed to avoid showing too much gold at the buccal

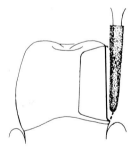

Figure 8.37 Reduction of the palatal surface, described as stage 1, removes undercut from this surface

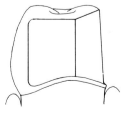

Figure 8.38 The second stage of preparation for a posterior partial veneer crown is the approximal reduction

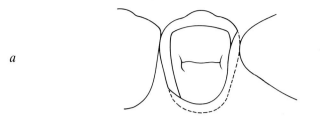

a

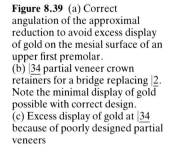

Figure 8.39 (a) Correct angulation of the approximal reduction to avoid excess display of gold on the mesial surface of an upper first premolar.
(b) |34 partial veneer crown retainers for a bridge replacing |2. Note the minimal display of gold possible with correct design.
(c) Excess display of gold at |34 because of poorly designed partial veneers

b

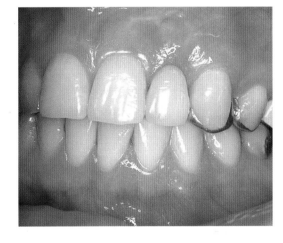

c

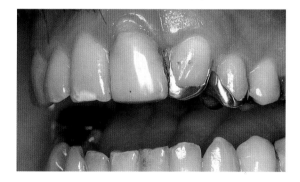

margins and should converge between 2° and 5° towards the occlusal surface (Figure 8.39).

3. Occlusal reduction. A cylindrical diamond at ultra speed or a wheel-shaped diamond at conventional speed may be used to make this reduction. The occlusal surface is reduced following the cuspal planes to allow complete coverage with 1 mm of gold wherever the opposing teeth meet the surface (Figure 8.40). Other areas need less reduction and 0.5 mm is generally sufficient.

Figure 8.40 In stage 3 the occlusal surface is reduced to allow coverage with 1 mm of gold

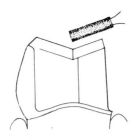

4. *Approximal grooves or boxes*. As has already been mentioned, much of the retention and stability of a partial veneer crown is derived from the approximal grooves. These must be in line with each other and the planned line of withdrawal. A tapered fissure bur is used to make these grooves. The bur is held against one approximal surface and a cut made to a depth of the radius of the bur. The second groove is then made on the other approximal surface, and finally, when their position and direction are satisfactory, both grooves are deepened to the equivalent of the diameter of the bur (Figure 8.41). Where there is insufficient room to prepare the grooves in this way they may be cut from the occlusal surface. This will minimize the danger of cutting adjacent teeth, but this is not an easy method for preparing the grooves in the exact direction required. They should finish gingivally, just within the finishing line of the preparation. It is generally wiser to prepare these grooves at low speeds to avoid the possibility of overcutting. They may be placed either centrally in the approximal surfaces or towards the buccal side (Figure 8.42). Central gooves are easier to place and provide adequate retention in most posterior teeth. They may be preferred to the longer buccally placed groove when there is an existing proximal restoration present.

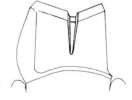

Figure 8.41 The preparation of approximal and occlusal grooves is described in stages 4 and 5

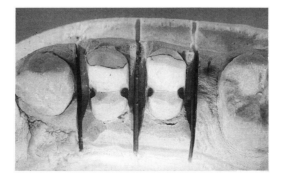

Figure 8.42 Dies of two upper premolar partial veneer crown preparations with centrally placed grooves

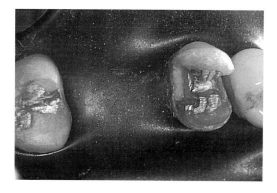

Figure 8.43 Box prepared in the distal surface of the anterior retainer for a fixed–moveable bridge

A box will always be required distally if the preparation is for the anterior retainer of a fixed-movable bridge, in order to allow room for the dovetail joint (Figure 8.43).

The treatment of caries. Caries which is not removed in the course of the standard preparation is excavated and replaced with a cement base if this can be covered by the proposed restoration. More extensive caries may require a full veneer crown.

Existing restorations. An existing restoration may be treated as if it were tooth substance provided there is no evidence of recurrent caries and that it can be covered by the new crown.

5. Occlusal groove. The mesiodistal fissure should be deepened with a cylindrical diamond or tungsten–carbide bur and this goove made continuous with the approximal grooves. It gives added rigidity to the casting and also increases resistance to displacement.

If there is any caries in the fissure it should always be cut out in this manner.

6. Finishing the preparation. The buccal margin of the occlusal surface is slightly bevelled and the cervical finishing line defined so that a minimum cavo-surface angle of 135° is produced (Figure 8.44).

It will be necessary to smooth the preparation to eliminate the rough surfaces left by the ultra-speed instrument. Any sharp angles on the preparation are also rounded and this particularly applies to the junction between the approximal and palatal surfaces.

The reverse bevel must be deepened on some lower teeth to provide

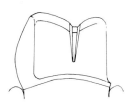

Figure 8.44 The completed preparation, showing rounded angles

Figure 8.45 Buccal view of a die of |5 showing reverse bevel extended down the buccal cusp beyond the region of occlusal contact

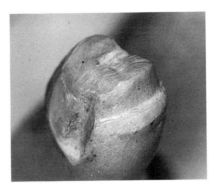

resistance to displacing occlusal forces especially in the presence of faceting (Figure 8.45).

Impression techniques and materials used are very similar to those used for full veneer crowns and are described in Chapter 5. The subject of temporary coverage is dealt with in Chapter 4.

Try-in, cementation and finishing

The routine for try-in, cementation and finishing a partial veneer crown is the same as that for a full veneer crown. Particular care should be taken to check the margins of the restoration and it is also essential to check that the occlusion is correct. Obvious high spots may be adjusted with the aid of thin articulating paper. After making the necessary modifications the crown is re-polished before cementation.

Chapter 9

Restoration of the space

Conventional bridges

General principles

After some experience with inlays and crowns, the knowledge already gained can be applied to bridges. Other principles have to be considered in addition to those underlying the restoration of a single tooth, and these are now discussed. For convenience of description, bridges will be considered in two main categories: conventional and resin-bonded (Figures 9.1 and 9.2). It will be seen that a well-planned and constructed bridge can restore the health and function of the masticatory unit. The plan should take into account not only the appearance and strength of a bridge, but the present and future health of the tissues involved.

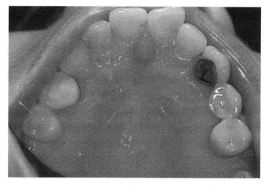

a

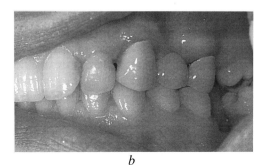

b

Figure 9.1 Occlusal (a) and buccal (b) views of a conventional bridge replacing an upper first premolar

Figure 9.2 A resin-bonded bridge
replacing a lower first molar tooth

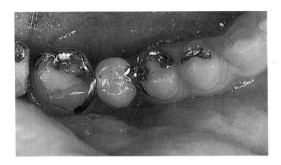

Indications and contra-indications

There are many indications for the construction of a bridge and only too
often the patient's wish to have a bridge rather than a denture is not
mentioned. However, there are, of course, many clinical reasons for bridge
construction, such as deterioration of the occlusion if a gap is left unfilled.
Teeth adjacent to the gap may drift and cause premature contacts, or loss of
contact, increasing food packing and the risk of caries. Loss of function is not
necessarily serious if the gap is small.

Although occlusal stability may initially be lost as a consequence of
extraction and non-replacement, tooth movement may result in an occlusal
relationship that is stable and acceptable from a functional viewpoint. In
cases of doubt, serial study casts will allow an assessment to be made as to
whether occlusal stability has been achieved. In some situations, orthodontic treatment will be required to re-align teeth or regain lost space before
bridgework. In these cases, the bridge may serve an additional function in
maintaining the result of the orthodontic treatment.

The improvement of appearance is an important reason for constructing a
bridge, and it must be made clear to the patient that few small bridges can
surpass the appearance of a well-constructed partial denture. However, the
comfort and stability of a bridge are generally much greater than even the
best removable appliance. Finally, a most important indication for a bridge
is based on the principle that all appliances in the mouth may cause damage
to teeth and periodontal tissues. Therefore, a bridge can be superior to a
denture because it covers less tissue and consequently has less potential for
periodontal damage. Replacement of missing teeth with partial dentures
may be a far more common source of periodontal disease than previously
considered.

The age of the patient is not important if there are overriding reasons for
the construction of a bridge. The very young patient is usually excluded from
consideration for a conventional bridge because of possible further tooth
movement and the size of the dental pulp, but bridges can and should be
constructed for dental and psychological reasons for young cleft-palate
patients. Wind instrument players require a lip seal that is difficult to achieve
with a partial denture in the anterior region of the mouth. For these patients
a bridge should, therefore, be considered even if the state of the dentition in
the posterior region is not ideal.

The clinical criteria that determine the advisability of embarking on bridge work must be judged on an individual basis. Consideration of these criteria at an early stage in treatment planning, and an assessment of the patient's ability to cooperate in the prevention of further dental disease, will avoid disappointment at a later stage.

As indicated in Chapter 2, efficient plaque control is essential for the long-term success of any bridge.

In preparing teeth for conventional bridgework, it is frequently necessary to remove substantial amounts of sound tooth tissue. The amount of tooth tissue to be removed may be greater than for individual crown preparations because mutual parallelism may be required between abutments that are out of alignment. Also, space may be required within the retainer contours for a moveable joint. The decision to provide a bridge must take these factors into account and the dentist must be convinced that the risk of pulp death is minimal before proceeding with treatment.

Definitions

In order to help the understanding of the following chapters, the main terms in use are defined (Figure 9.3).

Bridge   A dental prosthesis that is attached permanently to remaining teeth. It replaces a tooth or teeth and cannot be removed by the patient. Terminology sometimes differs between 'fixed bridge' for the above and 'removable bridge', which is a removable partial prosthesis.
Abutment   The tooth that supports a bridge, or part of a bridge, and to which a retainer is cemented.
Retainer   The terms 'abutment' and 'retainer' are frequently confused, but are not interchangeable. A retainer is that part of a bridge which is cemented to an abutment tooth, and in a conventional bridge, could be an inlay, full veneer crown or partial veneer crown. A retainer may be united to a pontic, another retainer or both.
Major and minor retainers   The retainer in a fixed-moveable bridge that is rigidly united to the terminal pontic is known as the 'major' retainer. A

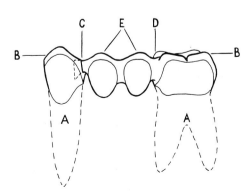

Figure 9.3 The components of a bridge. (A) Abutment tooth; (B) retainer; (C) moveable joint; (D) soldered joint; (E) pontics

retainer that is united to a pontic by a semi-rigid joint is called a 'minor' retainer.

Unit   Each part of the bridge, retainer or pontic may be referred to as a 'unit'. Therefore a bridge replacing one premolar and using two retainers is described as 'three-unit bridge'.

Span   The part of a bridge that covers the edentulous area is called a 'span'. It is connected or joined to retainers at both ends in most bridges, but only at one end in the case of cantilever bridges.

Pontic   Each individual tooth replacement in a bridge is termed a 'pontic'. A span may be composed of single or multiple pontics. A pontic is not always a reproduction of the tooth it replaces in the arch. If, for example, a space left by the loss of an upper first molar has closed, it may be replaced by a premolar pontic. The all-gold pontic frequently used to replace a missing lower first molar does not resemble a natural tooth except for the shape of the occlusal surface.

Pier   Any abutment other than the terminal abutments of a bridge may be called a 'pier'. 'Intermediate abutment' is probably a more descriptive term.

Joint or connector   These are synonymous terms used for the junction between any two units of a bridge.

Conventional bridges   These bridges employ conventional retained designs and do not depend on adhesive techniques for their retention.

Resin-bonded bridges   These depend on adhesive techniques for their retention and are cemented with resin cements.

Hybrid-bridges   These bridges consist of one or more conventional bridge retainers combined with a resin-bonded retainer.

Types of bridge

Fixed–fixed

In this type of bridge, all joints are either soldered or cast in one piece to connect, rigidly, all the abutment teeth. This type of bridge requires equal and good retention at either end of the edentulous span. Also it must be possible to produce mutual parallelism of all retainers.

Fixed–moveable

This form of bridge (sometimes incorrectly termed 'fixed-free') incorporates a stress-redistributing device (normally a slot and a dovetail), which allows limited movement at one of the joints between pontic and retainer. The 'fixed' end of the bridge has a rigid connector that is usually distal to the pontic. This is the major retainer. The minor retainer, which has the moveable joint, does not require as much retention as the major retainer. Because the abutment carrying the minor retainer can be depressed in its socket without the retainer being held rigidly to the rest of the bridge there is no need for full occlusal coverage with this retainer. The moveable joint will give full support to the pontic against vertical occlusal forces, and will allow limited movement in response to lateral forces (Figure 9.4). This prevents the movement of one retainer transmitting torsional forces directly to another and breaking the cement seal. The extension of an arm from the

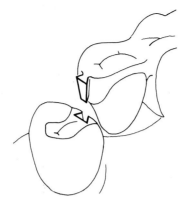

Figure 9.4 The dovetail joint or connector

pontic to an adjacent tooth does not constitute a moveable joint, and is in most cases merely an antirotational device. The 'cantilever' effect of the non-rigid design can place additional stress on the major retainer and, therefore, a strong abutment is required. This design may be contra-indicated for long edentulous spans.

Where there is a difference in the inclination of the abutment teeth and a common path of insertion cannot be prepared, a fixed–moveable bridge sometimes provides a solution to the problem.

Cantilever

A cantilever bridge has a pontic connected to a retainer (or retainers) at one end only. A disadvantage of this type of bridge is the leverage imposed on the abutment tooth. For this reason the abutments are often multiple, and the bridge is not used where the occlusal forces on the pontic will be heavy. The retainers must be joined rigidly and, therefore, as in the fixed–fixed bridge, they should be balanced for strength and retentive power. For example, if a partial veneer crown is joined to an MOD intracoronal inlay without coverage of the cusps, there is a danger that the cement seal of the MOD retainer will eventually fail.

A cantilever bridge is commonly used for the replacement of an upper lateral incisor from a canine. If the root of the canine is short or slender, rotation about its long axis may occur. This can be prevented by re-designing the pontic to provide some degree of wrap around the proximal aspect of the central incisor. If this tooth is unrestored then the patient must have excellent plaque control to reduce the risk of secondary caries. A fixed–moveable bridge is an alternative choice.

Spring cantilever

This bridge provides a method of supporting a pontic at some distance from the retainer. This type of bridge is both tooth and tissue supported. A gold bar, which fits in contact with the palatal mucosa, connects the pontic to the retainer (Figure 9.5). It provides a solution to the problem of replacing an upper central incisor when the anterior teeth are spaced. Upper premolars are the best abutments for replacement of an upper central incisor. Strong

Figure 9.5 A spring cantilever bridge replacing a central incisor. The abutments are the second premolar and the first molar

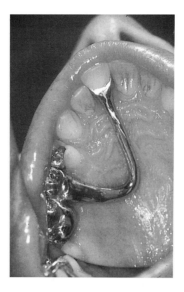

retention is required, as for all cantilever bridges, and double abutments are usually necessary. The connecting bar should follow a wide curve to provide additional mucosal support and limit adverse leverage. The bar should be oval in cross-section so that food passes easily over it.

The spring cantilever bridge is not an ideal prosthesis because of the area of mucosa covered permanently by the bar, and it should be used with discretion (Figure 9.6). It is not well suited to patients with a steeply vaulted palate and its use is rarely indicated in the lower arch because of the lack of suitable tissue support.

The retention of a spring bridge is severely tested when force is exerted in an apico-incisal direction, such as when the patient bites on sticky food and then opens the mouth. This movement tends to put the whole stress on the retainer at an angle that might destroy the retention. To avoid this weakness, two retainers in adjacent teeth are soldered together to give added strength. It is better to have the bar carried from the distal retainer to avoid the adverse lever effect caused by making the connection to the anterior retainer. The oral hygiene can be maintained remarkably well, using dental floss passed under the connector to clean beneath the bar.

Complex
A combination of any two or more of the above designs may be referred to as a complex or compound design.

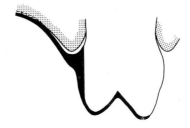

Figure 9.6 A cross-section of the palatal bar. The relationship of the palatal bar to the palate and the free gingivae differs

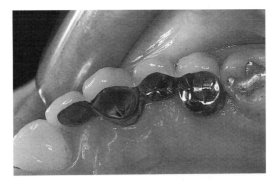

Figure 9.7 A 'complex' or 'compound' bridge using both fixed–fixed and cantilever designs

Variations in design

The basic designs already listed may be combined in a number of ways. Figure 9.7 illustrates a combination of a fixed–fixed design for the repalacement of the upper first premolar with a simple cantilever design for the replacement of the upper lateral incisor. As a general principle it is wise to use several small bridges to replace a number of missing teeth rather than replace them all with one large bridge. This will simplify replacement if a single unit fails (Figure 9.8a, b).

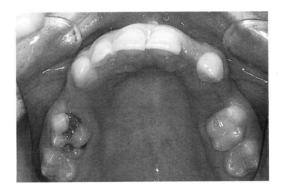

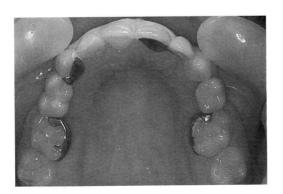

Figure 9.8 Three, small, resin-bonded bridges replacing missing teeth

Figure 9.9 Comparison of tissue coverage using various types of dentures and a bridge

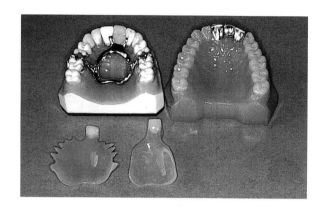

General considerations in bridge work

The patient

When explaining to a patient the differences between a bridge and a denture, the advantages of a denture must not be minimized and its economical advantage should not be forgotten. However, the disadvantages of a removeable denture with the large area of tissue covered, which needs to be maintained plaque-free, particularly at the gingival margins, must be mentioned and if possible demonstrated on a model. The display of clasps should also be demonstrated. Figure 9.9 shows how much tissue is covered by various types of dentures and the comparative freedom of palatal surfaces when a bridge replaces a denture.

The main advantage of a bridge is that it is fixed as part of the dentition and cannot be removed from the mouth. Furthermore, it usually involves only teeth adjacent to the space, so that plaque removal is comparatively easy. The lifespan of a bridge is often questioned by patients and the answer depends on many factors, such as the maintenance of good oral hygiene, control of periodontal disease and dental caries. It is not appropriate to quote a 'mean' lifespan taken from a survey of bridge failures.

The main disadvantages of bridge work are the time and cost involved, and the problems associated with repair after damage. Unless the patient understands the reason for the restoration, and is enthusiastic and likely to cooperate during tooth preparation, problems and misunderstanding may arise later.

Ideally the patient must maintain a high standard of oral hygiene and appreciate the necessity of good plaque control. Realistically, some compromise may be acceptable here but the periodontal condition has to be stabilized unless the patient is prepared to accept a reduced lifespan of the bridge.

The edentulous space

Bridges are ideally used for restoring small gaps within an otherwise complete arch having strong and well-supported teeth at either end of the space. If the vertical height of the space has been diminished by the overeruption of an unopposed tooth it is sometimes possible to reduce the tooth and produce a more favourable occlusal plane. However, a veneer crown may be necessary to cover the dentine exposed during the reduction of crown height. The space may also be diminished by drifting, rotating or tilting of the teeth that bound it. Correction of these malpositions may be advisable for several reasons:

1. When a tooth is tilted it is difficult to obtain a common path of insertion with other abutment teeth.
2. Tilted teeth usually have a diminished vertical height, at least on one surface, and therefore potential loss of retention. They are also difficult to prepare for a retainer, particularly a partial veneer crown.
3. If abutment teeth are prepared in their tilted position, periodontal problems are likely to occur between the abutment tooth and the pontic.
4. Removal of plaque becomes difficult when the interproximal spaces are not readily accessible.
5. In the case of mandibular molar tilting, orthodontic uprighting of such teeth is usually well-tolerated by patients and can make subsequent bridge construction more satisfactory.

The space available for the pontic is important, especially in the anterior region if the appearance is to be good. It may sometimes be increased by orthodontic means when there is room to move adjacent teeth. An alternative is to construct retainers that are narrower mesiodistally than the original abutment tooth. A narrow space can sometimes be restored to give a pleasing appearance by using an overlapping pontic design (Figure 9.10). This is a situation where a diagnostic wax-up can be particularly useful in planning the bridge. If the length of the span is too great for a normal-sized pontic, several possibilities must be considered, such as orthodontic treatment, wider retainers, or an alternative design, such as a spring cantilever bridge.

A midline diastema can create a difficult bridging problem. It may be possible to close the gap by orthodontic means, even at the cost of creating a space distal to the canines. This new space can then be bridged as part of an overall design, but other factors, such as the occlusion and number of posterior teeth, must be taken into account.

Occlusion
The abutment support and the amount of retention required vary not only with the length of the span, but also with the force exerted by the opposing teeth. This subject is dealt with in Chapter 3.

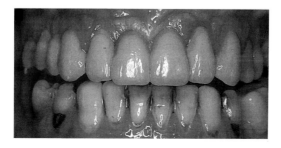

Figure 9.10 A six-unit bridge replacing the upper central incisors. The pontics overlap the lateral incisors because they could not be accommodated in the space available

Support and periodontal health

The abutment teeth must be able to provide support for a bridge, with all the extra leverage and torsion that it will impose. This support is related to the amount of root area secured in healthy bone. If the root area is insufficient or the bone has shown a resorptive reaction, there is a risk of the abutments becoming loose.

Deep, infrabony pockets or recession involving the bifurcation of the roots are contra-indications for their use as abutments in most cases. Some estimate of the future periodontal support can be gained by examining the periodontium and the radiographs. Gingival inflammation should be reduced by plaque control, so that no bleeding points exist, before bridge construction is started. A young patient with evidence of irregular bone loss is a poor choice for bridge work. Involvement of the furcation areas of molar teeth suggests a poor prognosis. The patient without furcation involvement who has little resorption of bone, which is mainly horizontal and evenly distributed, can be accepted for bridge work if plaque control can be achieved and signs of active periodontal disease eliminated.

Health of mucosa

Correct bridge design will allow the friction of mastication, toothbrush and interdental cleaners to act on the maximum area of mucosa and at the same time will prevent food-packing. This area of mucosal coverage can be kept to a minimum and should be accessible for cleaning with dental floss. All pontics have some area of tissue contact, except for the all-gold (so-called 'self-cleansing') pontic. When contact with the gingivae exists it should be minimal and without pressure, although an exception to the principle about gingival contact is the palatal bar of a spring cantilever bridge. This, apart from its ends where it joins retainers and the pontic, is recessed into the palate. Even with a well-constructed bridge the cooperation of the patient in keeping it clean is essential to ensure its long life.

Strength

The strength of the bridge is limited by the strength of its individual units. This is an obvious fact that is easily overlooked when concentrating on another aspect, such as appearance. The strength is largely dependent upon the materials used, which are discussed later. Points of potential weakness are joints, the gold frames or backings for pontics, and also occlusal or incisal surfaces. The requirements of strength for any individual bridge will depend on the amount of masticatory force it has to resist over the length of span and retainers. For example, a bridge opposed by a full denture has to resist much less occlusal force than one opposed by natural teeth.

Appearance

The problem of appearance with bridges becomes increasingly more important towards the front of the mouth. If the patient is prepared to show some gold, a more conservative choice of retainer design may be possible (either conventional partial veneer or resin-bonded). Metal ceramic crowns reduce the problem and can produce an excellent appearance, but in order to accommodate the metal frame and the porcelain veneer, considerable reduction is required on the labial aspect of the tooth. In situations where there is minimal occlusal stress an all-porcelain bridge can provide the best possible appearance. Such bridges should not normally exceed three units and failure rates may be high.

Occlusal function

Apart from the static function of maintaining the continuity of teeth in the dental arch and restoring appearance, a bridge should also improve the patient's chewing ability.

Abutment crowns

Crown size. A common cause of bridge failure is the choice of abutments with crowns that are too small to provide sufficient retention for the bridge. The clinical crown should have enough height to allow sufficient retention in the retainer preparation. Any tooth with less than 4 mm interproximal height from marginal ridge to gingival attachment is unsuitable for extracoronal retention. Pins or posts may be used for extra retention in the case of short crowns, but their use increases the difficulty of constructing the bridge. With a small tooth there is a greater danger of placing the pin-hole into the pulp chamber or outside the root. The main factors determining the amount of retention required in a given situation are: length of span; tooth or teeth to be replaced; design of bridge; occlusal function; and patient habits.

The longer the span, the greater the stress on the retainers and the greater the chance of their becoming uncemented. Replacement of a molar will require more retention than that for a lower incisor. Replacing an upper canine in a patient with a canine-guided occlusion will make more demands on bridge retention than for a situation where occlusal function on the pontic is restricted because of natural tooth guidance. This type of replacement may be an indication for converting the occlusion from a canine protected to a group function pattern (see Chapter 3).

Crown strength. Caries, existing restorations or endodontic treatment may have weakened an abutment crown, perhaps severely. The extent of the caries, either a primary lesion or secondary caries under a restoration, must be known before the type of retainer can be chosen. Failure to assess these points by clinical and radiographic examination before a bridge is started may involve the operator in a hasty change of design during the subsequent preparation. Minor undercuts, which do not involve the cavo-surface margin, can be obliterated with cement. Larger losses of tooth tissue are best restored with amalgam using pins for extra retention, and the whole covered by a veneer crown retainer. Root-treated anterior teeth will require a core retained by a post in the root canal.

Crown shape. The shape of an abutment crown may present retention problems and this is particularly so when dealing with short or conical teeth. Retention of this type of retainer depends mainly upon slots placed in the approximal surfaces, which should therefore be as long as possible.

Figure 9.11 Radiograph of a lower first molar, showing secondary dentine in the pulp chamber but a very long mesial pulp horn

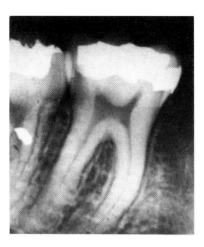

Pulp

The size of the pulp can be assessed from a radiograph and the operator's knowledge of pulp morphology. Secondary dentine formation is seldom symmetrical, and the preparation of a retainer may expose a pulp horn. The likelihood of such an accident can be seen particularly well in the lower first molar, where the mesiobuccal horn often remains large when the remainder of the pulp has diminished in size (Figure 9.11). A rotated or tilted tooth may have a relatively small pulp, which is nevertheless vulnerable because of the position of the tooth. This may be the case with a rotated upper lateral incisor or a tilted lower molar.

Clinical assessment of the state of the pulp is difficult in the absence of symptoms. If a positive response is elicited by an electrical pulp tester or bur, and no exposure of the pulp is present, it may generally be assumed to be healthy enough to receive a bridge retainer.

Elective endodontic treatment

Anterior teeth that have lost most or all of their coronal tooth structure will require endodontic treatment and the placement of a post and core. Endodontic treatment may also be required for malaligned or overerupted teeth to allow for a more favourable occlusion on the final restoration. Special consideration should be given to any tooth where caries has extended so deeply that the pulp may have become chronically inflamed. In these situations it may be wise to undertake elective endodontic treatment, with the proviso that this is carried out well before proceeding to preparation of the abutment tooth.

Endodontically treated teeth

There is no contra-indication to the use of a pulpless tooth as part of a bridge if there is a satisfactory root filling. On the other hand, a periapical lesion or other evidence of inadequate endodontic treatment should be reviewed because the extra stresses imposed by the bridge may cause further deterioration of the periapical tissues. A well-condensed root filling close to the apex and continuity of the apical bone can be taken as evidence of a satisfactory response to root canal treatment. The need to reinforce the clinical crowns of such teeth has been stressed in Chapter 8. A post and core is normally indicated as part of the restoration because these teeth will have lost a significant amount of coronal dentine support.

Abutments

Path of insertion
The inclination of the abutment teeth will determine the path of insertion of a bridge and may indicate that a fixed–fixed bridge is not possible. Lines drawn on a study cast will help determine the angulation of the long axes of the teeth (Figure 9.12).

Various paralleling devices are available (Figure 9.13a, b) and a simple surveyor is a useful aid in planning a common path of insertion on the study cast.

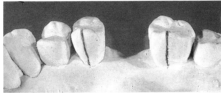

Figure 9.12 Lines parallel to the long axes of the premolar and molar teeth illustrate the divergence of inclination of the abutment teeth

Figure 9.13 (a) 'A simple parallelometer'. (b) A more elaborate parallelometer designed for use with an air-turbine handpiece

a

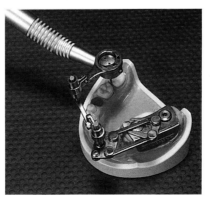

b

The approximal contours of the teeth adjacent to the abutments must also be considered to ensure that they will not interfere with the proposed line of insertion of the bridge. If the proposed abutment teeth are tilted from a common long axis the following points should be explored:

1. Can any other teeth be used as abutments?
2. Is the tilting too severe for the construction of a fixed–moveable bridge? If the long axes of the proposed abutment teeth differ by more than 20° an alternative design of bridge may be more suitable.
3. Can any improvement be made by orthodontic means, and would the patient tolerate this?
4. Would a cantilever bridge be possible?

Patients with gross misalignment of teeth are not usually a problem because preliminary assessment generally indicates their unsuitability for bridge work. In borderline cases it is helpful to prepare the abutments on a duplicate stone model and compare the final result with radiographs to determine possible pulpal involvement.

Retainers for conventional bridges

The same principles regarding pulp protection during preparation, design and marginal finish apply here, as they do for a single restoration.

The choice of retainers
Several types of retainers are available for use in bridge work, and their choice will depend on:

1. The retention required.
2. The amount of abutment crown available.
3. The strength of dentine remaining after preparation of the tooth.
4. The extent of existing restorations to be covered.
5. The amount of visible metal that will be tolerated.
6. The occlusal or incisal protection required.

The margins of retainers should be placed supragingivally wherever possible because a supragingival margin is healthier. Furthermore, the preparation, impression and fitting of the retainer are easier when working to a supragingival margin. However, it may be necessary for the sake of appearance to place those of anterior retainers within the gingival crevice on the labial aspect of an abutment tooth.

Types of retainers

Inlays, partial or complete veneer crowns, thimble or telescopic crowns, and intra-radicular posts are the available alternatives. The use of pins or posts with inlays or crowns will add to the retention.

Inlays
The use of intracoronal inlays without cuspal coverage is restricted to the minor retainer of a fixed–moveable bridge. Inlays without cuspal coverage

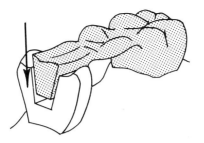

as the retainers in a fixed–fixed bridge often fail at the cement seal. The reason is that the abutment tooth can be depressed in the socket while the retainer is supported by the remainder of the bridge (Figure 9.14). This conflict of forces may cause the eventual fracture of the cement seal. The minor retainer of a fixed–moveable type is not connected rigidly to the rest of the bridge and is free to move in a vertical direction towards the alveolus. It must, however, have sufficient retention to withstand stresses from other than a vertical direction.

The MOD inlay with covered cusps is the least restoration that should be used as a major retainer of a fixed–moveable posterior bridge, or for either retainer of a fixed bridge.

Inclusion of approximal surfaces. Both approximal surfaces should be covered in major retainers. It is rarely possible to restore the damage caused by subsequent caries in an uncovered approximal surface of an abutment tooth without endangering the bridge.

Additional retention. The use of pins for additional retention in a Black's cavity requires great care to avoid penetration of either the pulp or the periodontal ligament. Buccal and lingual extensions, which project between the cusps onto the buccal and lingual surfaces, will add to the retention of this type of cavity in molars.

The posterior full veneer crown
This restoration is described fully in Chapter 8 and only those points relevant to its use as a bridge retainer are described here. Although a full veneer crown gives greater retention than a partial veneer crown, the appearance of these crowns is not always acceptable. In this case a metal ceramic crown may be used.

The partial veneer crown
This restoration is also described in Chapter 8 and only the points relevant to its use as a bridge retainer are discussed here.

When the proximal section of a partial veneer is to receive the male attachment of a moveable joint, sufficient room must be provided in the gold of that section for the dovetail slot to be cut. This is made possible by placing a box in the appropriate surface, in place of the usual retention slot.

Figure 9.15 Relative failure rates (%/year) of major bridge retainers. (After D. H. Roberts)

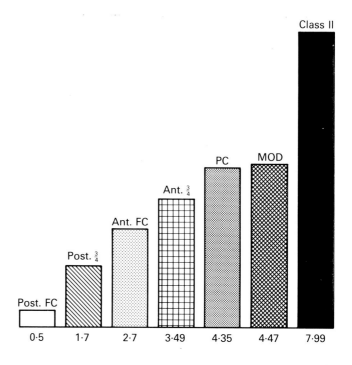

Telescopic crowns

This retainer is constructed in two parts: an inner open-topped sleeve made of hard gold, and an outer full crown to cover both the abutment crowns and the inner sleeve. This type of retainer is sometimes used to overcome differences in the inclination of abutment teeth, which cannot be resolved by the retainer preparations. It is the outer crown that is soldered to the other units. The amount of tooth substance that would need to be removed from the mesial surface of a tilted molar abutment to ensure a path of insertion for a fixed–fixed bridge will lead to loss of retention between the mesial and distal surfaces of the retainer. The use of a telescopic crown in these circumstances enables the mesial and distal surfaces to be prepared for one line of insertion (the inner sleeve) whilst the line of insertion of the bridge is reproduced on the outer surface of the sleeve (Figure 9.16). Because of the changed contour of the mesial surface of the tilted molar shown in Figure 9.16, particular attention must be paid to plaque removal in this area of the bridge. If additional retention is required for the inner sleeve, parallel buccal and lingual slots may be used.

The principle of telescopic crowns is used when constructing multiple unit bridges with fixed joints, as in a periodontal splint. The outer crowns are placed with a proprietary temporary luting cement because they may then be removed for inspection of the interdental papillae or even for repair.

Abutment roots

As an approximate basis for estimating the amount of support required, the combined root area of the abutment teeth should not generally be less than

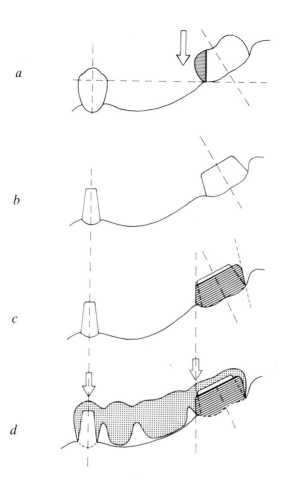

a

b

c

d

Figure 9.16 The use of the
telescopic crown for a fixed–fixed
bridge. (a) Shaded area shows the
amount of tooth to be removed to
allow insertion of a fixed–fixed
bridge. (b) Preparation of the
abutment teeth. (c) Telescopic
crown fitted to distal abutment.
(d) Fixed–fixed bridge fitted to
mesial abutment tooth and distal
abutment tooth with telescopic
crown. Telescopic crown retainers
are less commonly used now with
the improvements in fixed–
moveable designs

that of the teeth to be replaced. In 1926 Ante stated that: 'The combined
pericemental area of the abutment teeth should be equal to or greater in
pericemental area than the tooth or teeth to be replaced'. However, there is
now evidence that this statement is too rigid. The work of Nyman, Lindhe
and others has shown that the life of a bridge depends as much upon the
quality of periodontal support as its quantity. Furthermore, occlusal design
of the retainers and pontics to preclude undue stress on the periodontal
tissues is an important prerequisite. As general advice, however, it will be
seen from Table 9.1 that a canine may be an acceptable abutment for a
lateral incisor, but a lateral incisor will not be suitable to carry a central
incisor. The figures also illustrate the wisdom of using two premolar
abutments when replacing a canine in a canine-guided occlusion.

The number, length and shape of the roots will indicate the amount of
support available for the bridge. As a general rule the preference for
abutment support is given in the following order: Upper 6 7 3 4 5 1 2, Lower 6
7 3 5 4 2 1. Third molars may be used as abutments, but exhibit such variation
of form that it is difficult to place them in any order of preference.

If only half of the root length is in bone, the effective loss of support for
that tooth is greater than half, because the root tapers towards the apex.

Table 9.1 Mean areas (mm^2) of the roots of upper and lower teeth. (After D M Watt)

Upper teeth	Central incisor	205
	Lateral incisor	177
	Canine	267
	First premolar	220
	Second premolar	217
	First molar	455
	Second molar	417
	Third molar	305
Lower teeth	Central incisor	162
	Lateral incisor	175
	Canine	272
	First premolar	197
	Second premolar	204
	First molar	450
	Second molar	400
	Third molar	373

Each case should be assessed separately and not by any rule of thumb. The area of root needed for support will depend on the length of the span. Upper anterior bridges frequently have a forward projection, which creates a leverage arm and therefore requires additional abutment support (Figure 9.17).

If roots are small and tapered they will provide less resistance to the extra masticatory forces imposed on a bridge span and it will be necessary to overcome this problem by increasing the number of abutments. On the other hand, roots that are flattened or oval in cross-section offer more resistance to rotation than those that are round. Molars with divergent roots offer greater resistance to movement than those with fused roots.

When the bifurcation or trifurcation of a posterior tooth is exposed by gingival recession it may be unsuitable for a bridge abutment. However, in some instances the environment in the furcation region can be controlled, especially with the aid of endodontics and root resection. The remaining

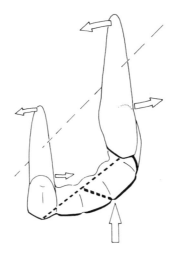

Figure 9.17 Additional leverage due to an upper anterior bridge projecting beyond the major abutment teeth may require compensation by the addition of further abutment teeth, especially if the arch is curved; in this case, the two first upper premolars, which are not shown in the diagram

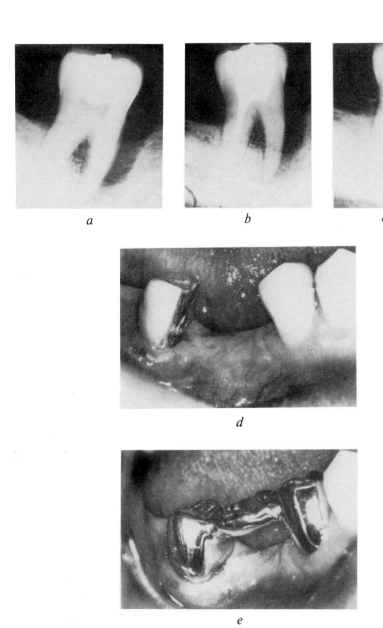

a   *b*   *c*

d

e

Figure 9.18 (a) Bifurcation involvement of lower right second molar. (b) Root filling in distal root. (c) Hemisection undertaken. (d) Three months after hemisection. (e) Completed bridge

root or roots can then be used as a bridge abutment is periodontal health is restored (Figure 9.18).

Multiple abutments

Occasionally teeth adjacent to a gap are potentially weak abutment teeth and their sole use as the mesial or distal abutment tooth for the bridge is contra-indicated. This is usually found in patients where periodontal disease has reduced the bony attachment of the tooth. In such circumstances extra retention in the form of an additional abutment tooth is required. The 'weak' abutment tooth is therefore splinted to the other abutments, and will not have to bear all the occlusal forces.

Pier abutments

The failure rate of pier or intermediate abutments may be higher than that of terminal abutments. This is due to flexing of the span of the bridge or differential tooth movement under load. Where very large bridges are to be made it is generally preferable to design these as several short bridges, which may or may not be inter-connected, rather than making a very large single bridge. Therefore, if a failure of any component should occur, it is only necessary to remake the section containing the failed component rather than replacement of the whole bridge.

Bone surrounding abutment teeth

Radiographs of the abutments should be scrutinized to observe the amount of bone present and its continuity, especially around the apices of the abutment roots. Occasionally unsuspected areas of radiolucency will be found on one root of a molar that has given a positive reaction to pulp tests. The examination of any other dubious teeth in the arch is included at the same time, because, although not involved in the bridge, their loss may indicate a change in treatment plan.

Pontics

Pontic design and selection are among the most important parts of bridge design and cannot be related to previous experience of inlay and crown work.

Pontic form

Whatever type of pontic is chosen, it should conform to several basic principles of design if the bridge is not to become an area of stagnation and a source of infection. Pontics should be aesthetically pleasing and be adequate functional replacements for lost teeth. They should be non-irritating to the mucosa and allow effective plaque control.

Occlusal surfaces

In order that the span can be functional and yet prevent excessive occlusal forces damaging the abutments, the occlusal width of pontics is kept within the boundaries formed by straight lines connecting the buccal and lingual surfaces of the abutments (Figure 9.19). The width of the occlusal surface should not be narrowed beyond that of the tooth being replaced. The assumption that reducing occlusal width reduces occlusal forces and creates conditions more favourable to the periodontium of the abutment tooth has not been proven.

Figure 9.19 (a) Shaded area showing limits of occlusal surface that the pontic must not exceed. (b) Invaginations are made in the occlusal surface of the pontic so that buccal and lingual embrasure spaces are maintained to help plaque control

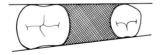

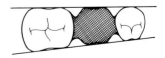

a   *b*

There is considerable evidence that damage attributed in the past to occlusal trauma is caused primarily by dental plaque. Therefore, facilitating plaque control should be a primary aim of pontic design. Nevertheless, trauma, which causes the tooth to move in more than one direction (jiggling trauma), should be avoided as this will act as an important secondary factor in speeding the destruction caused by existing periodontitis. Buccal and lingual/palatal invaginations (embrasures) are therefore placed at the junction between any two units of the bridge. The angles of these invaginations are kept wide and rounded for ease of cleaning.

Buccal and lingual or palatal surfaces

The buccal and lingual or palatal surfaces should lie in approximately the same plane as the surfaces of the adjacent teeth if they are to gain the maximum benefit from the cleansing effect of the cheek, lips and tongue during mastication. For the same reason they should also be slightly convex.

Angle of contact. The angle formed by the junction of these surfaces of the pontic with the gingivae must be kept as wide as possible to discourage food stagnation (Figure 9.20a, c). This rule is often overlooked in the effort to reduce the amount of pontic area in contact with the gingivae, thus producing an acute angle between pontic and mucosa and a food-trapping area (Figure 9.20b).

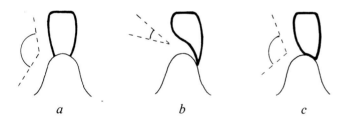

a *b* *c*

Figure 9.20 The relationship of pontic to ridge. (a) This is a ridge lap pontic. The mucosal contact area covers approximately the root area of the missing tooth. (b) Line contact. The acute angle forms a food trap. (c) This is a modified ridge lap pontic and it removes the concave mucosal contact area

Area of contact. The lines where the buccal and lingual surfaces of the pontic join the mucosa should be as close to one another as possible, thus covering the minimal area of mucosa.

Unfortunately this ideal is not always possible, because where the buccal line of junction is visible it must conform closely to the cervical margins of the adjacent teeth. A sudden change in the line of the cervical margins of a row of teeth is immediately noticeable, and should be avoided where possible.

Loss of the outer alveolar plate will often necessitate a rather sharp curve from the buccal surface to the cervical margin. This is the one departure from the rule requiring a wide angle of contact between the outer face of the pontic and the mucosa. Even in this case the angle of contact should be kept as wide as possible (Figure 9.21b, c).

Mucosal surface

Plaque must be removed from the tissue contacting surface of a pontic regularly to maintain tissue health. In the mandibular posterior region,

Figure 9.21 (a) The cervical margin of the central incisor pontic is at a different level from those of the adjacent teeth. (b) The broken line indicates the type of alveolar bone loss that may take place in the upper incisor region. (c) The shaded area shows minimal tissue contact with resorbed alveolus. The labial face of the pontic is in the same plane as the adjacent teeth. (d) This indicates the slight concavity that can seldom be avoided on the tissue surface of the pontic. (e) When there has been excessive loss of alveolus, the fitting surface of the pontic must be redesigned as shown, and the patient instructed in the need for special cleansing at the gingival margin

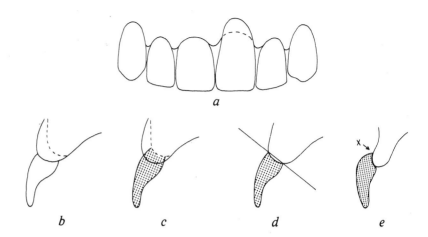

where appearance is not normally a problem, a simple solution is to use pontics that do not contact the mucosa and have a smooth, rounded undersurface. These are called sanitary (or hygienic) or wash-through pontics (Figure 9.22). Properly finished, such a pontic does not interfere with normal occlusion and speech, and it is easy to keep clean with dental tape or interproximal brushes. In all other regions of the dentition, for aesthetic reasons, pontics should make light contact with the alveolar mucosa. This mucosal contact should be to firmly attached gingivae without any hyperplastic tissue. If the edentulous ridge, that the pontic will contact, is irregular in shape with hyperplastic tissue, then gingival recontouring should be undertaken and the tissue allowed to heal before placement of the bridge.

With a well-designed bridge the pontic should barely touch the labial aspect of the ridge for a distance that is dictated by aesthetics as well as allowing space for the interdental papilla (Figure 9.23). The naturally occurring convex ridge shape leads to a concavity on the tissue surface of a

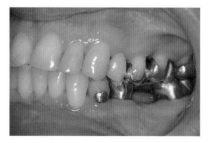

Figure 9.22 A lower all-gold bridge with a 'sanitary' pontic

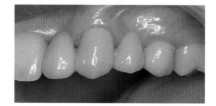

Figure 9.23 A four-unit metal–ceramic bridge replacing the lateral incisor and first premolar. There is some excess cement interdentally, which needs to be removed

ridge lap pontic, which may prevent plaque removal by flossing. The labial contour of the pontics should match as far as possible the neighbouring teeth. The tissue surface should be polished to a high gloss and be accessible for plaque removal by the patient. A common mistake is to make the interproximal spaces too narrow, resulting in poor access and gingival hyperplasia. It is important that interproximal joints are convex, well-rounded, and easy to clean.

The material of which pontics are constructed appears to be of lesser importance than correct pontic design, which is essential to enable the patient to keep the area plaque-free. It is important that the area adjacent to the edentulous ridge be convex or flat so that the patient can clean it with dental tape or floss. In practice, there may be a slight concavity of the surface, which cannot be avoided (Figure 9.21d). The pontic should be in contact with the soft tissue without causing blanching and the edges should be slightly rounded to avoid irritation. Detailed reproduction of the indentations in the mucosal contour is not required and would only encourage the accumulation of plaque.

Embrasures

The space between the units will, in some cases, be determined by the pontic and retainer used. The interdental space should be accessible to cleansing by dental floss or single-tufted brushes (Figure 9.24). Narrow spaces, which will encourage capillary attraction and subsequent stagnation, are better closed completely. All parts of the interdental surfaces should be curved, so that they are accessible from either side. Particular attention should be paid to the interproximal spaces in the posterior regions. Adequate spaces are most important there because of the larger buccolingual width of these teeth and poor access makes cleaning difficult.

The most useful cleaning devices that a patient can use are interdental brushes and dental floss or tape. Floss, particularly if used with a threader, or Superfloss (Educational Health Products Inc., New Canaan Conn., USA), which has a stiffened end for easy interproximal insertion, is often successful.

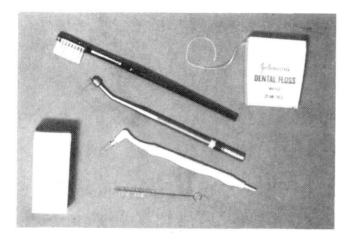

Figure 9.24 Various cleaning devices

Brushes are available in many different shapes, sizes and forms. Each patient has to find the brush that is comfortable and of most assistance with a particular bridge, and no one brush could be claimed as the 'best'. The dentist should assist in the choice. Much depends on the manual dexterity of the patient and on a willingness and ability to use the device regularly.

Types of pontic

Although there are many types of pontic, all of them except one represent an attempt to solve the problem of combining the mechanical properties of gold with the appearance of porcelain. The choice of pontic will depend partly on the material chosen for the retainers, the vertical space available, the appearance and angulation of the abutment teeth, and the ridge form. Metal–ceramic pontics are frequently used in both anterior and posterior regions. A limited number of pontics will be listed in order of common usage at present. There are others, but many of the proprietary pontics are not readily available.

The all-gold pontic

This pontic is used to replace molars where appearance is not important. There is no mucosal contact and sufficient space is left between the gold and mucosa to avoid stagnation. The occlusal surface is given cuspal form and the mucosal surface is made slightly convex so that every point can be reached from the buccal and lingual aspects for cleaning with toothbrush and dental floss. The joints with other units are rounded on the mucosal surface, which is achieved during soldering.

Metal–ceramic pontic

The metal–ceramic pontic is suitable when the retainers, or at least one of the retainers, are made of the same material. It has the advantage that the tissue contact is porcelain and that cervical and occlusal staining can give the pontic a very lifelike appearance. In the anterior region the provision of a translucent incisal tip is relatively easy. The bonding of the porcelain to the gold produces a pontic of great strength and there is little chance of the porcelain fracturing.

Pontics for spring cantilever bridges

These usually take the form of a porcelain jacket crown cemented to a core/diaphragm assembly at the terminal end of the connecting bar. This design avoids having the pontic/cement junction next to the mucosal surface.

Joint or connector

The connector, sometimes called the joint, is that part of the bridge that joins a retainer to a pontic, or one retainer to another. The connector can be rigid, usually referred to as fixed, or it can be semi-rigid, usually referred to as moveable (Figure 9.25).

Fixed. As the name implies, this is a rigid joint between two units of the bridge and allows no movement between the units. As this provides the

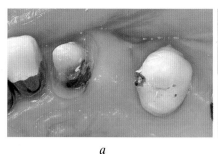 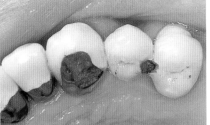

a   *b*

Figure 9.25 (a) The distal retainer of a three-unit bridge with the female section of a moveable connector. (b) The anterior section of the bridge in place

maximum strength for a bridge, the fixed connector is the one most commonly used. In the past all fixed joints or connectors were soldered but now, especially when alloys for bonding porcelain are used, several retainers and pontics of a bridge may be cast as one piece. It is necessary to have a sufficiently large surface area for the connector to avoid fracture at this, potentially the weakest, part of the bridge. However, it is also necessary to leave sufficient room for a healthy dental papilla.

Moveable. There are many ways of providing a joint that allows limited movement between pontic and retainer as opposed to the rigidity of the soldered joint. Some of these can be constructed in the laboratory but there are many prefabricated moveable joints or 'precision attachments' with various eponymous names.

The moveable joint recommended for the newcomer to bridge work is a simple dovetail male-and-female attachment. It is easy to construct with the materials available in the average laboratory. The disadvantage of this joint is that it can be withdrawn in an occlusal direction.

The construction of a dovetail moveable joint must be visualized when the abutment teeth are being prepared, and enough space allowed for the slot to be cut in the gold of the minor retainer. The slot must be in the same line of withdrawal as the major abutment. This joint functions because it has only one line of withdrawal in an occlusal direction and allows only imperceptible movement in other directions. The longer and narrower it is, compatible with strength, the better it will function. These considerations are easily overlooked when preparing a tooth for the minor retainer that is to contain the slot.

The retainers are cast, finished to a satin surface, and fitted to the model. A vertical cut is started in the minor retainer by a fine, flat fissure bur, in line with the path of withdrawal of the major retainer. Before this is deepened, a check should be made to determine whether the slot will lie entirely in gold. The initial cut is then increased to the full depth that is safely allowed by the thickness of the gold. At this depth the cut is widened to form a dovetail with a slight longitudinal taper. The internal angles can be sharpened by the use of an inverted cone bur along the length of the slot, remembering that a wax pattern will be required to reproduce the slot accurately.

The wax pattern of the slot is then taken as an integral part of the pontic frame and both are cast in one piece. Alternatively the moveable joint can be cast from a commercially available burnt-out pattern (Sterngold Mini-Rest). See Figure 9.25.

Resin-bonded bridges

A resin bonded bridge consists of a cast metal framework that is cemented with composite resin to abutment(s) which have had preparation(s) confined to enamel.

Direct composite bonding techniques may be used to provide short-term replacement of missing teeth either with natural tooth crowns as pontics, or with acrylic or composite pontics. The limiting factor is the weakness of the composite resin 'connector'.

Flexible wire mesh, proximally-placed orthodontic brackets and pins placed into the interdental resin have all been used in attempts to increase the life of these restorations.

General considerations

Resin-bonded bridges were originally used for the replacement of anterior teeth in young patients where conventional bridge work was contra-indicated because of pulp size, crown length or patient management. These patients often have sound abutments, but inadequate plaque control and little experience of operative dental treatment. Many of them participate in contact sports, and removable partial dentures have often been the 'compromise' solution adopted in spite of their potential adverse effect on periodontal health. Therefore, resin-bonded bridges became the preferred treatment. They were used as an interim or temporary prosthesis. Little, if any, enamel preparation was undertaken and the technique was essentially 'reversible'.

The resin-bonded bridge is now an accepted permanent alternative to the conventional bridge. Definite tooth preparation is frequently necessary to improve retention and assist in location. It is particularly suitable for the treatment of patients who have unrestored, caries free, abutment teeth and short edentulous spans. It may simplify a complicated treatment plan by serving as an intermediate restoration, eliminating the need for a remove-able prosthesis. Other indications for their use as an interim restoration include patients with a mixed or periodontally compromised dentition.

Indications

1. Where abutment teeth have satisfactory appearance.
2. Where suitable space exists for an aesthetic pontic.
3. Where sufficient enamel surface area is available for bonding.
4. Where abutment teeth are not heavily restored. The proximal and lingual surfaces of the abutments should normally be free of caries or large restorations.
5. When adequate occlusal clearance of $\geqslant 0.5$ mm can be achieved without exposing dentine.
6. When posterior occlusion is stable and abutment(s) protect pontic during functional movements of opposing teeth.
7. As interim replacements where expense, uncertain prognosis or both contra-indicates other treatment.

8. Resin-bonded bridges may also be used for multiple units.
9. Where an unusually large surface area of enamel is available for bonding.
10. When periodontal support for abutments is similar and abutment teeth are firm.

Contra-indications

1. When it is not possible to obtain good isolation by rubber dam technique.
2. Insufficient enamel; short, small or heavily restored abutments.
3. Mobile or hypoplastic abutment teeth.
4. Severe tooth wear/parafunctional activity.

Resin-bonded bridges are a fairly recent development and they have sometimes been used in inappropriate situations leading to failures. All the clinical and laboratory procedures associated with the planning, construction and cementation of a resin-bonded bridge are as critical as with a conventional bridge in order to ensure success. Whilst a resin-bonded bridge may be a conservative restoration for selected patients there is a high risk of failure in unsuitable cases and careful patient selection is very important.

Bridge design

Fixed–fixed, fixed–moveable, cantilever and spring cantilever designs have all been used with resin-bonded bridge work. Debonding of one retainer of a fixed–fixed design will not result in immediate dislodgement. However, this type of failure is relatively common with this design because of differences in retainer coverage and retention combined with variations in periodontal support and occlusal loading. Single abutment cantilever and fixed–moveable designs have a higher success rate and the simple cantilever should be the design of choice wherever possible. This design produces less torsional stress on the composite lute. If debonding of a cantilever bridge occurs, the patient will seek treatment immediately. Unilateral debonding of a fixed–fixed design may, however, lead to rapidly progressive caries under the debonded retainer before the patient seeks treatment. The minor retainer of a fixed–moveable design must contain a positive rest for the non-rigid connector. A dimple or V-shaped rest is sufficient to prevent facial rotation (Figure 9.26). A tapered box-type rest seat is recommended for posterior use. This design allows independent tooth mobility, while decreasing dislodging forces on the abutment casting. The pontic is supported during function but is free to separate in the unseating direction. Such bridges may be used successfully even in long-span situations (Figure 9.27).

Hybrid bridges
Resin-bonded retainers may be used in combination with conventional retainers when fixed–moveable connectors are employed (Figure 9.28). This is known as a hybrid bridge. If a rigid connector is used with this combination of retainers, cementation is complicated by the need for different cements,

Figure 9.26 (a) The rest recess on the palatal surface of the central incisor, which is a fixed–moveable retainer, is clearly visible. The outline for the retainer on the canine can also be seen. (b) The assembled bridge

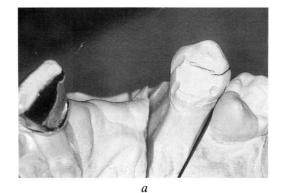

a

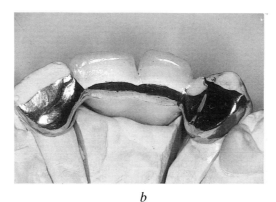

b

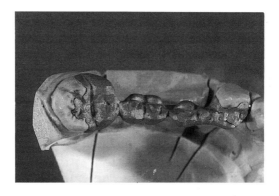

Figure 9.27 The metal framework of a long span fixed–moveable bridge. The rest seat is in the distal part of the premolar retainer

Figure 9.28 A four-unit hybrid bridge replacing a premolar. There is a moveable joint in the second premolar and the anterior retainer is resin-bonded. The gold crowns are splinted because of periodontal destruction. Normally the second premolar would suffice as the minor retainer

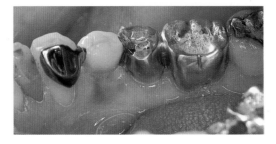

and the risk of retention failure is increased. This is because of the differential retention of the two types of retainer and the lack of occlusal cover normally found with resin-bonded units.

For hybrid fixed–moveable bridges, the resin-bonded retainer should normally be made the major retainer. Therefore, debonding will not require replacement of the conventional retainer and it is easier to create room for a moveable joint within the confines of a conventional retainer. Placing the joint extracoronally in the pontic section is not advisable as the lever arm created increases the risk of failure.

Resin-bonded vs. conventional bridges

The resin-bonded bridge is a highly conservative restoration involving minimal tooth preparation restricted to the enamel of the abutment. Preparation time is only a few minutes per retainer. No anaesthesia is required because of the lack of dentine involvement, which also eliminates the risk of pulpal irritation. There is no risk of soft tissue trauma because of the supragingival finishing line to the preparation. This simplifies impression taking as gingival retraction is seldom required. There is usually no need for a provisional restoration. However, it is not possible to alter the shape, size, colour or position of the abutment teeth as may be done with conventional bridge work; pontic space also cannot be altered.

It is frequently not possible to assess the need for occlusal adjustment until after the bridge has been cemented. Cementing or 'bonding' is more technique-sensitive than for a conventional bridge and requires considerably more time.

Metal/resin retention methods

Table 9.2 summarizes the various metal/resin retention mechanisms.

Macromechanical retention

The development of the 'Rochette bridge' was a significant advance as it combined the advantage of resin-bonding with the strength of a cast-metal retainer. The Rochette design has composite/metal retention by perforations in the metal framework backing (Figure 9.29). Retention is limited, the framework is weakened, and the composite lute is exposed to the oral environment. Rochette bridges are indicated for:

1. Immediate replacements.
2. Interim replacements.

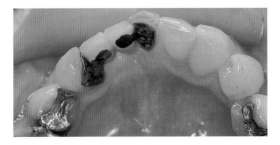

Figure 9.29 Two cantilever Rochette bridges

3. Adolescent patients.
4. As part of a complex treatment plan (during periodontal/endodontic treatment).
5. Uncertain prognosis.
6. Risk of trauma (contact sports).

Mechanical retention

Mesh wax patterns are difficult to adapt and cast completely but will provide good retention (Figure 9.30). Macroretention is created on the retainer fit surface by using salt crystals to obtain voids in acrylic resin patterns. It provides good retention, no special apparatus is required, any alloy may be used and framework retention may be readily assessed. These techniques require increased retainer bulk. In the Crystalbond technique a combination of soluble and insoluble particles in a soluble gel vehicle are applied to the stone die just short of the retainer margins before the Duralay resin pattern fabrication. The retainer is then soaked in water to dissolve away the gel and the soluble particles. The pattern is invested and cast; the undercut areas of the framework fit surface are visible as positive projections or negative depressions in the framework (Figure 9.30b).

Micromechanical retention

Grit blasting (50–250 micron AlO) of the framework fit surfaces will produce a roughened retentive surface, which may assist macroretention techniques or may be used with chemically-active composite resin cements. In the latter situation the retention is both mechanical and chemical (microchemical).

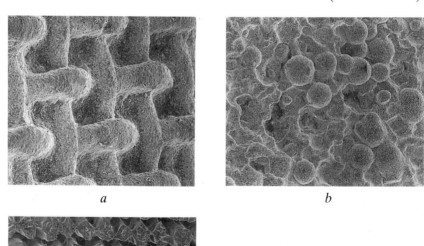

a   *b*

c

Figure 9.30 Scanning electron microscope views of a resin-bonded retainer fit surface. (a) Mesh retention. (b) Crystalbond retention. (c) Electrolytically-etched retention

Table 9.2 Retention techniques

Retentive mechanism	Examples
Macromechanical	Rochette
Mechanical	Mesh Retention (e.g. Duralingual) Salt Crystals Beads & Crystals (e.g. Crystalbond)
Micromechanical	Grit blasting Electrolytic etch Chemical etch
Microchemical	Chemically-active resins (e.g. Panavia Ex; Super-Bond C & B; C & B-Metabond) Alloy surface treatments (e.g. Tin plating, Silicoating)

Electrolytic etching of non-precious alloy can produce micromechanical retention via surface porosities akin to acid etching of enamel (Figure 9.30c). Composite resin will flow into the porosities and polymerize to form resin tags. The non-fit surface of the bridge has to be masked with wax before etching and special laboratory apparatus is required for electrolytic etching. Chairside electrolytic etching machines have been developed, which simplify the process as the surfaces not to be etched do not require masking with wax (Figure 9.31).

Nickel–chromium and cobalt–chromium alloys are the most commonly used because the nickel–chromium–beryllium alloys, which etch best, are not considered safe for routine laboratory use. There is no reliable chairside method for checking the adequacy of an etched surface. Chemical etching techniques have been introduced to simplify the process. However, the hydrofluoric acid gels are caustic and therefore extreme care is required with their use. They should be kept well away from the clinical area.

Microchemical retention
Certain adhesive resin cements bond to grit-blasted (non-precious), oxidized or tin-plated precious alloy surfaces.

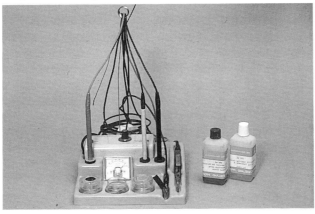

Figure 9.31 A chairside electrolytic etching apparatus

These chemically active composite resin cements form chemical bonds to the oxidized surfaces of non-precious alloys. Two effective materials are (1) Panavia Ex (Kuraray Co., Japan), which contains an active phosphate ester of BIS-GMA in the monomer, and (2) Super Bond (Morita, Japan) or C & B Metabond (Parkell, USA; Ventura, UK), which contain 4-META as the active chemical agent in the resin. Contamination of the grit-blasted surface must be avoided before cementation as this may seriously impair the metal/resin bond. Contaminated surfaces are difficult to clean effectively. Chairside grit-blasting units allow metal surface treatment between the try-in and cementation. The fit surface of the bridge is sand-blasted with 50 micron AlO. The cement is mixed according to the manufacturer's instructions and in the case of Panavia Ex the retainer margins are covered with Oxyguard in order to prevent oxygen inhibition and incomplete polymerization of the cement.

The micromechanical retention gained from the grit-blasted surface may be increased by tin-electroplating the alloy surface. This results in a chemical bond between the tin and the retainer surface. The deposition of tin particles on the casting surface increases the surface area available for micro-mechanical bonding with composite resin. Precious-metal alloys may be tin-electroplated, which makes the technique more versatile than metal/ composite bonding techniques, which only bond effectively to non-precious alloys. There is no advantage in tin plating a cobalt–chromium alloy before cementation with Panavia Ex as simple grit-blasting will yield a better bond. The reverse is the case with precious alloys.

An alternative technique for chemical bonding is based on the adhesion of resins to silane bonding agents. A very thin, glass-like layer is built up on the roughened metal inner surface of the bridge using a Silicoater (Kulzer) apparatus. Silane is then coated onto this surface to provide a chemical link between the resin cement and the glass-like layer. The thickness of the two layers is less than 1 μm, and does not interfere with the seating of the casting. The silicoated surface has to be protected with an opaquer layer or a layer of resin if the bridge is not to be cemented within 30 min of silicoating.

Techniques based on chemical bonding of resins to metal alloys have many attractions. The use of adhesive resins simplifies laboratory procedures. It reduces expense because frameworks for chemical bonding are generally easier and quicker to prepare than those for mechanical retention. Also a wider range of alloys may be used in comparison to alloys

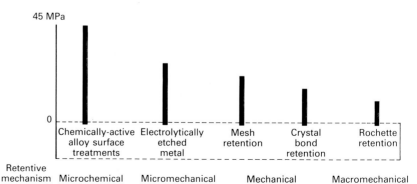

Figure 9.32 Mean tensile bond strengths (MPa) for several metal resin bond techniques (data summarizes the results of several investigations)

amenable to etching, and the total area of the inner surface of the framework is available for bonding.

The authors recommend either the silicoating technique for treating the fit surface of non-precious alloy resin-bonded bridge retainers or alternatively grit-blasting of the alloy fit surface and bonding with a chemically-active resin cement. Truly adhesive luting agents and microchemical retention mechanisms may eventually render macromechanical or micromechanical (etching) techniques obsolete.

Figure 9.32 summarizes the relative retentive values of the major metal–resin bonding techniques.

Table 9.3 Summary of advantages and disadvantages of metal/resin-bond mechanisms

Mechanism	Advantages	Disadvantages
Macromechanical retention (e.g. Rochette)	Simple technique No special equipment required Use any alloy Easy to remove Good appearance	Limited retention Bulky framework needed Composite lute exposed
Mechanical retention (e.g. Mesh)	No special equipment required Use any alloy Moderate to good retention Framework not perforated Retention site easily assessed	Increased retainer bulk Reduced retentive area Laboratory process difficult
Micromechanical retention (a) Electrolytically (b) Chemically etched	Good retention Thin framework Framework not perforated Whole area retentive	Etch is alloy specific Special apparatus needed Retention may be unreliable Difficult to evaluate etch Extra visit required Possible problems with appearance
Microchemical retention (a) Chemically-active resins (b) Alloy surface treatments	Good retention Whole area retentive Framework not perforated One visit, simple technique	Very good bond possible but alloy and surface treatments are critical Meticulous attention to detail required Long-term efficacy uncertain

Abutment tooth preparation

Tooth preparation improves the retention of resin-bonded bridges by increasing the contact area of enamel available for bonding and by reducing functional stresses on the composite resin lute. It also provides increased occlusal clearance and creates a positive seat for the restoration during try-in and bonding.

Guidelines for anterior preparations

1. Reduce palatal enamel by about 0.5 mm to produce adequate inter-occlusal clearance in all functional mandibular excursions. Less enamel reduction is required for mandibular teeth.

Figure 9.33 The approximal grooves on the canine retainer compensate for the limited circumferential retention

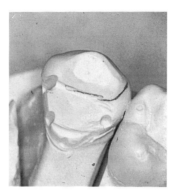

2. Extend the reduction incisally within 1–2 mm of the incisal edge and as far as functional and aesthetic considerations permit (see Figure 9.26b).
3. Extend gingivally to 1 mm from gum margin.
4. Extend proximally (adjacent to the edentulous space) as far as appearance permits.
5. Extend proximally (opposite to the edentulous space) to within 1 mm of the contact area.
6. Provide a cingulum rest to aid resistance form.
7. Use proximal grooves as substitutes for labial wrap circumferential retention (Figure 9.33).

Guidelines for posterior preparations
1. Replace any small proximal amalgam restorations with composite and/or glass ionomer cement.
2. Reduce proximal and lingual/palatal axial surfaces to provide a >180° 'wrap-around' effect and increase enamel bonding surface (Figure 9.34).
3. Produce knife-edge finish proximally to avoid dentine exposure (Figure 9.35).

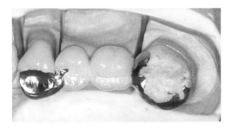

Figure 9.34 The posterior resin-bonded retainer of this bridge has 'wrap-round' retention

Figure 9.35 (a) The master cast of this small resin-bonded bridge has guide plane reduction and approximal knife edge finishing lines. (b) The bridge has rest seats and a 'wrap-round' design

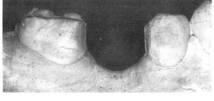

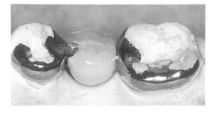

a   *b*

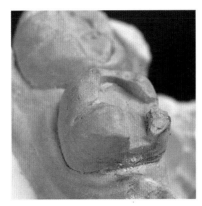

Figure 9.36 The cast of a lower molar mesio-occluso-lingual preparation. This tooth has a preexisting MO restoration

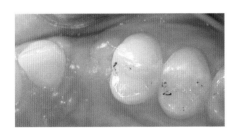

a

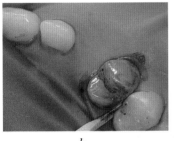

b

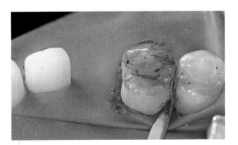

c

Figure 9.37 (a) The areas of contact on the premolar are marked with articulating paper. (b) Varnish is applied to the tooth to preserve the contact marks during preparation. (c) The completed preparation of the premolar for a resin-bonded retainer

4. Produce occlusal coverage for mesially tipped molars and for lingual cusps of mandibular first premolars to provide additional bonding area (see Figure 9.27). This is to supplement loss of bonding surface area from short teeth (Figure 9.36).
5. Use shallow proximal boxes or grooves (in enamel or restorative material) to assist retention and to compensate for the lack of circumferential retention.
6. Make occlusal rest seat preparations (Figure 9.37).

Impressions and temporary restoration

Temporary restorations are rarely required for teeth prepared for resin-bonded bridge work. In the anterior region a small amount of light-cured composite resin may be acid-etched to the opposing tooth/teeth to prevent overeruption while the bridge is being made. Impression techniques are dealt with in Chapter 5.

Try-in and cementation

Perforated framework (Rochette bridges) are cemented with a chemically-cured conventional particle size composite. Cements for other types of resin-bonded bridge are summarized in Table 9.4. Etched or silicoated bridges should have the retainer fit surfaces protected with a thin layer of light-cured, unfilled resin in the laboratory in order to prevent contamination at the try-in stage.

Table 9.4 Examples of suitable alloy/surface treatments/cement combinations

Alloy	Surface treatments	Luting resin
Nickel–Chromium	Grit blast	Chemically-active resin cement*
	Silicoat	Dual-cured† or chemically-cured‡ resin-bonded bridge cement
	Etched	Dual-cured† or chemically-cured‡ resin-bonded bridge cement
Cobalt–Chromium	Grit blast	Chemically-active resin cement*
	Silicoat	Dual-cured† or chemically-cured‡ resin-bonded bridge cement
Gold–Palladium	Grit blast/tin plate	Chemically-active resin cement*

* For example, Panavia Ex (Kuraray) or C & B-Metabond (Parkell).
† For example, Microfill Pontic C (Kulzer).
‡ For example, Comspan (Dentsply) or Nimetic Grip (Espe).

Try-in and cementation procedures

1. Clean the prepared teeth with a slurry of pumice and water, rinse and dry.
2. Try-in the bridge to check the fit, contour and path of insertion.
3. Place a rubber dam, allowing sufficient slack in the edentulous region for the bridge to seat passively (Figure 9.38).
4. Protect adjacent teeth with matrix strips before the abutment(s) are acid-etched (30 sec), rinsed (20 sec), and dried until the characteristic frosted appearance is visible (Figure 9.39).
5. Apply mixed bonding resin of a chemically-cured or dual-cured luting composite to the etched enamel and blow thin. Apply the mixed luting

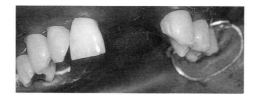

Figure 9.38 The rubber dam is placed with slack to allow the pontics to seat passively

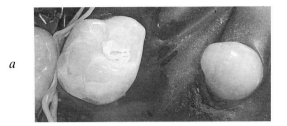

a

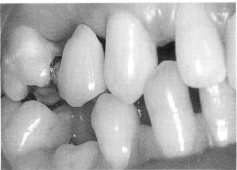

b

Figure 9.39 (a) The second premolar will be replaced by a cantilevered two-unit resin-bonded bridge. The molar abutment preparation has been acid-etched. (b) The fitted bridge

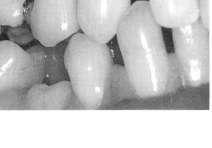

Figure 9.40 Duralay resin was used as a seating matrix to assist in the location of a Rochette bridge at the cementation stage

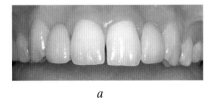

a

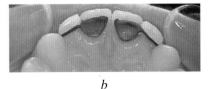

b

Figure 9.41 (a) The labial view of two small cantilevered resin-bonded bridges. (b) The palatal view of the same two small bridges

composite (either chemically- or dual-cured) to the fit surfaces of the retainers before seating the bridge into place. Duralay resin seating matrices (Figure 9.40) are useful for cantilever designs. Seating lugs, which form part of the retainer casting and lip over the incisal edges of the abutments, may be a useful alternative.

6. Maintain seating pressure while removing any gross excess of composite with a brush that has been dipped in resin. If a dual-cured composite is used, the retainer lute margin may now be light-cured. Maintain seating

pressure until the composite resin has set. If Panavia Ex cement is used to cement a grit-blasted non-precious alloy bridge then the barrier agent (Oxyguard), supplied by the manufacturer, should be applied to the margins after removal of excess cement.

7. Excess cement can be removed from the margins with a suitable hand and/or rotary instruments.
8. Check carefully for any cement remaining interproximally or cervically before removing the rubber dam.
9. Check the occlusion and adjust if necessary to ensure there are no premature contacts on the bridge in any functional occlusal position.
10. Final finishing of the resin/metal margin (using water-cooled burs) is best left until 1 week after cementation.

Examples of bridge design

Bridge design has been discussed in general terms, and some examples are listed a guide. For any situation there is frequently a considerable number of designs that could, theoretically, be used, but full consideration of all the relevant factors will generally indicate that many are unsuitable. It is not intended to suggest that the examples given below are the only designs suitable for the situations listed but they represent basic designs that may be helpful to consider before seeking a more complex solution. A design is often chosen because the operator prefers to use it, while the choice of retainer is sometimes dictated by the extent of existing restorations or the material chosen for the bridge. Furthermore, one-piece castings are often preferred to soldered joints. The designs are listed in order of the authors' preference and, wherever possible, simple designs have been chosen.

Joints that are either soldered, or form part of one-piece castings, are referred to as fixed. Bridges with multiple abutments may have a fixed joint between a distal abutment and a pontic, as well as a moveable joint between a pontic and a mesial abutment. The following abbreviations are used in the tables:

C = conventional	R = resin-bonded	H = hybrid
FF = fixed–fixed	FM = fixed–moveable	P = pontic
Ca = cantilever	SC = spring cantilever	

Tooth absent	Type of bridge	Design of bridge	Abutments	Distal retainer	Mesial retainer	Comments
2̲	C or R	Ca	3̲	Metal–ceramic crown or resin-bonded retainer	—	
2̲	C or R	Ca	1̲	—	Porcelain or metal–ceramic crown	All porcelain bridges are only suitable when the occlusion is light in all excursions of the mandible
2̲	C	FF	3̲ 1̲	Metal–ceramic crown	Metal–ceramic crown	
2̲	C, R or H	FM	3̲ 1̲	Metal–ceramic crown or resin-bonded retainer	Metal–ceramic crown or resin-bonded retainer	
2̲	C	SC	5̲ 4̲	Partial veneer or metal–ceramic crown	Partial veneer or metal–ceramic crown	A spring cantilever design is suggested only for patients with a natural space between the anterior teeth, where the occlusion is relatively light and where the palate is relatively flat and with firm mucosa. An implant is another possibility
1̲	C or R	FF	2̲ 1̲	Metal–ceramic crown or resin-bonded retainer	Metal–ceramic crown or resin-bonded retainer	
1̲	C	Ca	3̲ 2̲	Metal–ceramic crown	Metal–ceramic crown	
1̲	R	Ca	1̲	—	Resin-bonded retainer	
1̲	C or R	SC	5̲ 4̲	Partial veneer crown or resin-bonded retainer	Partial veneer crown or resin-bonded retainer	See comment above about choice of spring cantilever design
1̲|1̲	C	FF	(3) 2̲|2̲(3)	Metal–ceramic crown	Metal–ceramic crown	In suitable cases the canines need not be involved
1̲|1̲	C	Ca	3̲2̲| |2̲3̲	Metal–ceramic crown	Metal–ceramic crown	Two separate cantilever bridges
|1̲2̲	C or R	FF	1̲|3̲	Metal–ceramic crown or resin-bonded retainer	Metal–ceramic crown or resin-bonded retainer	
2̲1̲|1̲2̲	C	FF	(4) 3̲|3̲ (4)	Metal–ceramic crown	Metal–ceramic crown	The premolars are needed only where load is heavy
1̄	C or R	Ca	1̄ or 2̄	Metal–ceramic, porcelain or resin-bonded retainer	Metal–ceramic, porcelain or resin-bonded retainer	
1̄	C	FF	1̄|2̄	Metal–ceramic crown	Metal–ceramic crown	
1̄|1̄	C	FF	2̄|2̄	Metal–ceramic crown	Metal–ceramic crown	
1̄|1̄	R	Ca	2̄| |2̄	Resin-bonded retainer	Resin-bonded retainer	Two separate cantilever bridges
2̄1̄|1̄2̄	C	FF	(4)3̄|3̄(4)	Metal–ceramic crown	Metal–ceramic crown	The number of abutment teeth required depends on the occlusion and curvature of the arch
2̄	C or R	Ca	3̄	Metal–ceramic crown or resin-bonded retainer	—	
3̲	C or R	Ca	(5)4̲	Metal–ceramic crown or resin-bonded retainer or partial veneer crown	Metal–ceramic crown or resin-bonded retainer or partial veneer crown	Second premolar generally needed only in canine-guided occlusion. Not resin retained if canine-guided occlusion

Tooth absent	Type of bridge	Design of bridge	Abutments	Distal retainer	Mesial retainer	Comments
$\underline{4}$	C or H	FM	$\underline{5\ 3}$	Metal–ceramic crown	Class III inlay or resin-bonded retainer	The distal retainer and pontic are cast in one piece and the joint between the mesial retainer and the pontic is a slot and dovetail moveable joint
$\underline{4}$	R	FM	$\underline{5\ 3}$	Resin-bonded retainer	Resin-bonded retainer	A simple rest seat is incorporated into the $\underline{3}$ retainer
$\underline{4}$	C	Ca	$\underline{65}$	Metal–ceramic or full gold crown	Metal–ceramic or full gold crown	
$\underline{5}$	C	FM	$\underline{6\ 4}$	Partial veneer crown	Partial veneer crown or inlay/onlay	
$\underline{5}$	R	Ca	$\underline{6}$	Resin-bonded retainer	—	
$\underline{54}$	C	FM or FF	$\underline{6\ 3}$	Full gold crown	Metal–ceramic crown	
$\underline{6}$	C, R or H	FM	$\underline{7\ 5}$	Full gold crown or resin-bonded retainer	Partial veneer crown or resin-bonded retainer	A rest seat is incorporated into the $\underline{5}$ retainer
$\underline{6}$	C	FF	$\underline{7\ 5}$	Full gold crown	Metal–ceramic crown	
$\underline{654}$	C	FF	$\underline{7\ 3}$	Full gold crown	Metal–ceramic crown	
$\overline{4}$	C	FM	$\overline{5\ 3}$	Metal–ceramic crown	Partial veneer crown	
$\overline{4}$	C or R	Ca	$\overline{6\ 5}$	Partial veneer, metal–ceramic crown or resin-bonded retainer	Partial veneer, metal–ceramic crown or resin-bonded retainer	
$\overline{5}$	C, R or H	FM	$\overline{6\ 4}$	Full gold crown or resin-bonded retainer	Partial veneer crown or resin-bonded retainer	
$\overline{5}$	R	Ca	$\overline{6}$	Resin-bonded retainer	—	
$\overline{6}$	C, R or H	FM	$\overline{7\ 5}$	Full gold crown or resin-bonded retainer	Partial veneer crown or resin-bonded retainer	One of the few situations where an all gold 'wash through' pontic is frequently used
$\overline{65}$	C	FF	$\overline{7\ 4\ 3}$	Full gold crown	Metal–ceramic crowns	Three retainers are generally required to support these teeth
$\overline{65}$	C	FM	$\overline{7\ 4}$	Full gold crown	Metal–ceramic crown	
$\overline{54}$	C	FM or FF	$\overline{6\ 3}$	Full gold crown	Metal–ceramic crown	
$\overline{64}$	C	Complex	$\overline{7\ 5}$	Full gold crown	Metal–ceramic crown	$\overline{6}$ is replaced as a fixed unit, while $\overline{4}$ is cantilevered. This is not suitable where the premolars are heavily stressed
$\overline{64}$	C	FF	$\overline{7\ 5\ 3}$	Full gold crown	Metal–ceramic crowns	

General comments. In cases when some bridge units are made of metal–ceramic and others are made of gold, the metal–ceramic units are usually a one-piece casting and the gold units are soldered to them. Adhesive bridges may frequently be split into two cantilevered units, which will minimize the risk of caries developing under an undetected de-bond. Adhesive designs should not be used for complex designs. Hybrid bridges should be split into fixed–moveable units.

Chapter 10

Treatment planning and clinical case histories

The clinical procedures for bridge construction may differ but should always conform to the basic principles that have been outlined in previous chapters. These principles must be followed in planning and constructing any bridge.

Assessment of patient

It is important to encourage patients to explain their personal wishes and requirements, particularly about anterior bridges where appearance is of primary concern. This discussion will also provide an opportunity to assess the patient's ability to cooperate with prolonged treatment and lengthy sessions in the dental chair.

It is generally accepted that all routine treatment should be completed before bridge work is begun, and this early treatment will be an important part of the assessment of the patient.

Clinical examination

The clinical examination of the mouth should follow a set pattern. It should be an examination of the whole mouth and include an exploration of carious teeth, the periodontal condition of the whole dentition and radiographic examination. Radiographic examination of the whole mouth is in many cases essential. All too often it is limited to the area in which the bridge is to be constructed, with the result that a pathological condition in other areas, which might influence the planning, is not detected. In some cases orthodontic movement of proposed abutment or opposing teeth may be advantageous.

The level of oral hygiene and plaque control must be assessed. If it is unsatisfactory, instruction is essential and unless the patient understands the important role oral cleanliness plays in preventing further dental disease, a bridge may be contra-indicated. In many cases a considerable time elapses between the first examination of the patient and the start of the bridge construction. It is during this time that the patient can demonstrate a willingness and ability to cooperate in developing a good oral hygiene technique.

Study casts

Study casts are important before a bridge is planned. The articulated casts will help the operator to evaluate the angulation of prospective abutment teeth and the forces that will act against these teeth and the pontic. In many cases they serve as a useful guide for the technician and must be retained as a record of the pre-operative condition, to be referred to, if the need arises.

Investigation of existing restorations
The preliminary examination may reveal existing restorations in suitable abutment teeth. These restorations must be examined carefully, and if there is any doubt about their integrity, strength, condition of the pulpal floor or recurrent caries, they should be replaced.

Bridge design
Bridge design has been discussed in a previous chapter. There may be more than one design that could provide a satisfactory bridge. The chosen design is often a personal preference of the operator and made after consultation with the patient.

Consultation with the patient and appointment planning
The patient's main interest lies in the appearance of the finished product. The patient is not usually interested in the intricate problems of occlusal harmony or retention. However, if these problems demand, for instance, that a certain amount of gold will be visible, this should be explained. Furthermore it is helpful to explain the nature of the bridge to be made and the additional burden cleaning it will demand. Casts of bridge work will assist with this. The fact that certain teeth may have to be reduced or crowned must be explained. Finally, the patient must be given an estimate of the time and cost involved.

If possible, the appointments should be planned so that preparations are completed in one visit if the bridge is not large. In the case of a simple bridge replacing one tooth the impression can sometimes also be taken at this visit and the bridge cemented at the next visit. It is advisable to make a further appointment for a final examination.

Preparation of the opposing arch
Modification of the opposing teeth may be necessary and defective restorations in teeth of the opposing arch must be investigated.

Minor adjustments of the occlusal surfaces of opposing teeth are carried out at this stage. In some instances, where an opposing tooth has over-erupted into the bridge space, considerable reduction may be necessary. Any defective restorations must be renewed before bridge preparation. This may require a restoration to protect the cut surfaces of the tooth.

The notes on occlusal adjustment in Chapter 2 are as relevant to bridge construction as they are to the construction of crowns and inlays.

Clinical procedures

The clinical procedure in bridge construction, consists of the following stages: (1) preparation of abutments; (2) abutment impressions; (3) registration of the occlusion; (4) shade taking; (5) temporary coverage; (6) retainer try-in and localizing impressions; (7) trial fitting of bridge; (8) cementation of bridge; and (9) final examination of completed bridge.

Preparation of abutments

The preparation of the abutment teeth is described in earlier chapters. With extensive bridges it is advisable to rehearse the preparations on the study casts and then after the bulk of the tissue is removed in the mouth an alginate impression is taken. The new cast is surveyed; this makes it easier to determine the precise modifications necessary to complete the preparations.

Abutment impressions

Before impressions are taken, preparation of the gingivae and isolation of the teeth are necessary. The smallest amount of moisture present at the wrong moment can ruin an otherwise perfect impression. There is no rule with regard to the impression materials used. Elastic impression materials are used by most operators and the choice should be governed by the knowledge of the properties of the material, the clinical condition in which it is to be used and the skill developed by the operator and the dental surgery assistant in the successful use of a material.

In spite of careful gingival preparation and moisture control a perfect impression is not always obtained first time. Therefore, when planning the appointments, sufficient time must be allowed for a repeat impression should this be necessary. It is wise for impressions to be taken at a separate visit after the preparations are completed unless the bridge is a very simple one.

Registration of occlusion

Registration of the occlusion is important if a bridge is to function correctly. The techniques for recording the occlusion are described in Chapter 3.

Shade taking

The shade should be taken and checked during the procedures, preferably with colour-matched fluorescent or halogen quartz lighting.

Temporary coverage

Temporary restorations are important for protecting the abutment teeth, and their construction and fitting are decribed in the chapters on anterior and posterior crowns.

The ideal temporary restoration for a bridge, when the preparation of all abutment teeth has been completed, is a one-piece bridge made of acrylic resin. If the retainer preparations are completed at separate appointments, temporary crowns may be used. An existing denture may be used to maintain the gap. The temporary bridge is prepared either by the technician from a duplicate study cast or it is made at the chairside. Although chairside construction is time-consuming, it is sometimes a useful expedient.

Laboratory-made temporary bridges usually have a good appearance, are well tolerated by patients, save surgery time and are accurate. They are not as strong as gold but can be used for many weeks, although the bridge should be completed as soon as possible.

Retainer try-in and localizing impressions

Separate retainers may be tried-in and examined for fit, contact with the adjacent teeth and occlusion with opposing teeth before a localizing impression is taken. The larger the span of the bridge the more important this stage becomes. When bonded porcelain is used and the bridge consists of many units the subframe should be tried in before the addition of porcelain. However, many operators who have a good reliable working relationship with a technician dispense with the trial fitting of the metal subframe and have the porcelain added for completion without the intermediate stage.

Trial fitting

At the trial fitting care must be taken to remove temporary cement and debris. Some patients prefer a local anaesthetic for this, especially when the prepared abutments are exposed to cold air for prolonged periods. The bridge is then seated and the fit checked systematically. The retainers are examined for fit, occlusion and contact with adjacent teeth, while the pontics are examined for form, occlusion and contact with the mucosal surfaces. The contact area between pontic and soft tissue is examined carefully for excessive tissue blanching or free space between the pontic and the tissues. If either is seen, the pontic will have to be corrected. Finally, the general appearance, form, length of teeth and shade are checked. For this, one must step well back from the patient and observe the mouth and teeth while the patient talks, smiles and is in rest position.

Before final cementation it is important for the patient to have adequate time to examine the bridge with the help of a hand mirror and to make comments. At this point the patient has an opportunity to mention any problems and the dentist has the opportunity to explain, if necessary, that minor problems such as slight lisping usually disappear after some weeks. With large bridges a 24-hour try-in without cementation is recommended. Very slight movement can allow the bridge to seat more accurately on its abutments. It also gives the patient and relatives an opportunity to observe and comment on the bridge while away from the surgery environment. However, such a prolonged trial fitting is not always practicable, but it is sometimes possible to fit the bridge without cementation in the morning and ask the patient to return to the surgery for cementation later the same day.

If a bridge made of gold does not seat properly, a joint is cut and the retainers are then tried in separately. If satisfactory, a new localizing impression is taken for resoldering.

If a bonded porcelain bridge does not seat, the best solution is to remake the whole bridge; reheating of the metal subframe for alterations and then the addition of new porcelain layers cause technical problems and the porcelain may fracture from the bridge in a comparatively short time after cementation. Then, or course, it has to be removed and remade with great inconvenience to the patient and the dentist.

Cementation

Before the cementation of a bridge the abutment preparations must be perfectly clean and dry. The retainers are filled with cement and the preparations are also covered with a small amount of cement. Where pins are used some cement is placed into the pin-holes with a probe.

The bridge is seated by digital pressure and held firmly in place with a suitable instrument. In the case of a posterior bridge, after the initial setting of the cement, a cotton-wool roll is placed on the occlusal surfaces of the bridge and the patient is asked to bite firmly in centric occlusion. When the cement is hard, excess is removed with a probe and dental floss is passed under the pontic to remove any debris. Finally, the occlusion is rechecked.

Final examination

At a subsequent visit the occlusion of the bridge is examined. Burnish marks do sometimes appear due to 'high spots' and these must be adjusted to correct the occlusion. The gingival health is checked and the patient instructed in any further oral hygiene procedures necessary.

Illustrations of the clinical procedures

The bridges made for several patients are described to illustrate briefly the clinical procedures involved.

Case 1. *Immediate replacement Rochette bridge*

The patient had extensive untreated periodontal disease. The upper left lateral incisor tooth had recently been lost and the right central incisor tooth had very deep pocketing and required urgent extraction (Figure 10.1a). The long-term prognosis of the adjacent teeth could not be determined until thorough periodontal treatment, including possible surgery, had been carried out over several months. It would have been possible for a denture to be used but this may have increased the periodontal problems.

An immediate replacement Rochette bridge was therefore indicated. No

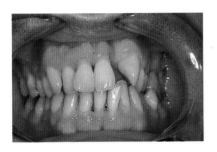

a

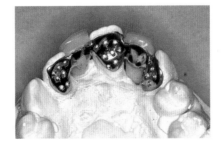

b

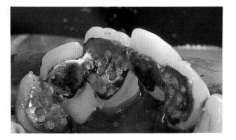

c

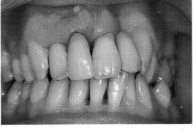

d

Figure 10.1 (a) Patient after initial oral hygiene instruction. The right central incisor tooth requires immediate extraction due to extreme bone loss. (b) The Rochette framework on working model showing retentive design. (c) At cementation, care was taken to ensure complete flow of the composite resin. Careful polishing and removal of excess was carried out. (d) Completed bridge in place. (Note blood at margins from extraction socket)

tooth preparation was carried out and an accurate impression taken. The central incisor to be extracted was sectioned from the working model and a Rochette framework made (Figure 10.1b).

To bond the framework into place, the incisor tooth was first extracted and a rubber dam placed to prevent contamination of etched tooth surfaces with blood from the socket. A conventional chemically-cured composite resin was used for cementation, care being taken to ensure that material had fully extruded through the retentive holes (Figure 10.1c).

A further advantage of the Rochette design in this case was that it could be easily removed later during treatment for access and then re-cemented.

Case 2.   A simple bridge replacing a first lower molar where appearance is not important (Figure 10.2)
This patient, aged 37, had a relatively low caries rate but unfortunately had $\dfrac{5\,|\,6}{6\,5\,|}$ extracted in childhood. Plaque control was good.

Her main complaint was of food packing between the upper molars on the right side. On examination, there had been drifting and tilting of the upper teeth and the upper right first molar had overerupted into the space created by the loss of the lower teeth on that side.

It was decided to provide an all-gold fixed–fixed bridge.

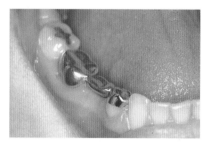

Figure 10.2 The illustration shows the bridge and inlays 14 years postoperatively

The occlusal surface of the upper right first molar was first reduced and other minor occlusal adjustments made in order to facilitate restorations.

Full crown preparation was undertaken on the lower right second molar and partial veneer crown preparation on the lower right first premolar with considerable protection of the buccal cusp. An all-gold bridge was constructed and fitted. Gold inlays were made for the upper right molars to restore the contacts between these teeth.

Case 3.   Replacement of the four lower incisors (Figure 10.3)
The patient was involved in a car accident causing, amongst other injuries, the fracture of the four lower incisors. On examination the canines were found to be non-vital.

Bridge design. It was decided to use a fixed–fixed design with the canine and first premolar on each side as the abutments.

Preparation. Endodontic treatment of the canines was completed and a post and core was fitted to each. The incisors were extracted and a temporary

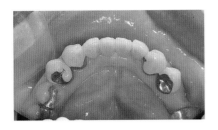

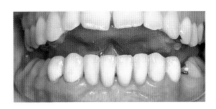

Figure 10.3 A lower anterior metal–ceramic bridge replacing the four incisors. The retainers are full crowns on both canines and first premolar abutments

bridge was made, using the canines as the abutment teeth. In view of the slight lingual tilt of the first premolars, it was relatively easy to prepare two full crown preparations on these teeth, which were near-parallel to each other. After some weeks to allow healing to take place the temporary bridge was removed, and an impression of the four abutment teeth was taken, using an elastomer as the impression material. An eight-unit bridge of bonded porcelain was then fitted.

There was a suspected fracture of the apical third of one canine root. Radiographic examination of the root after 3 months showed nothing abnormal. Should an apicectomy be required in the future, it could be carried out without hazard to the bridge.

Case 4. Replacement of missing incisor teeth with a resin-bonded bridge following ridge augmentation (Figure 10.4)
The patient had lost |12 traumatically with resulting loss of labio-palatal alveolar bone. A resin-bonded bridge had been provided but had repeatedly debonded due to insufficient retention because of the small retentive wings. This bridge utilized a flange attached to the pontics, which gave a poor appearance and made cleaning impossible (Figure 10.4a).

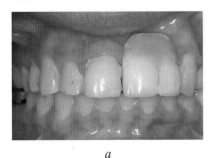

a

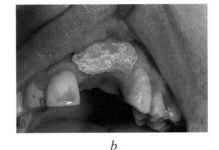

b

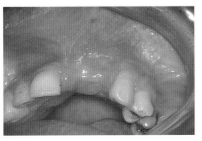

c

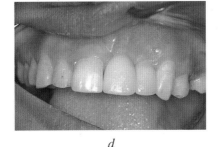

d

Figure 10.4 (a) Failed resin-bonded bridge with fixed gingival flange. (b) At surgery a block of bone substitute is shaped to rebuild the contour of the ridge. (c) Six weeks later following healing. (d) The completed bridge in place. (Note the normal length pontics)

The alveolar ridge was first rebuilt using hydroxyapatite based material (Proplast: Unitec Corp., USA). This is non-resorbable but is only useful in non-load bearing areas. A flap is raised and the material carved to bulk out the ridge as desired (Figure 10.4b), the aim being to allow for normal length and shape pontics.

Alternative ways of dealing with this situation include the use of gum-coloured extended pontics, false gingival prosthesis or removable bridge work based on milled bars, which can include flanges. All of these alternatives are very much compromises and best avoided if possible. If large amounts of ridge are missing a denture with a flange normally gives the best result.

Six weeks after healing (Figure 10.4c), the implant was considered stable and a new resin-bonded bridge was provided ensuring substantial bonding areas to minimize the risk of future debonding (Figure 10.4d).

Case 5.   Replacement of a lateral incisor by a bridge in a unilateral cleft palate patient, after creating a space for a pontic (Figure 10.5)
The creation of a space for a pontic required orthodontic treatment.

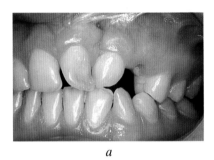

a

Figure 10.5 Crowning of a rotated central incisor with retraction of the canine and replacement of the lateral incisor. (a) The rotated central incisor adjacent to the unilateral alveolar cleft. (b) Palatal view showing the mesial drift of the canine. (c) Retraction of the canine and temporary crowning of the central incisor. (d) A four-unit metal–ceramic bridge replacing the lateral incisor. (e) Palatal view of the bridge showing the full cover of porcelain and occlusal staining on the premolar retainer

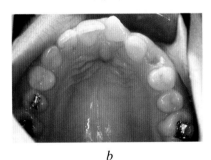

b

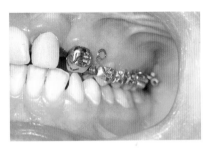

c

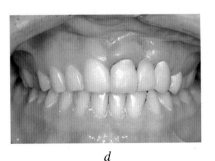

d

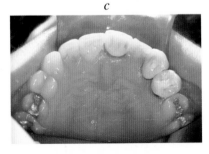

However, since prolonged orthodontic treatment is often resisted by adults, it was decided to devitalize and crown the central incisor and confine the orthodontic treatment to the retraction of the canine.

A unilateral fixed orthodontic appliance was used to retract the canine and create a space sufficient for a normal-sized lateral incisor.

In the meantime the central incisor was devitalized, root filled and a post and core was prepared and cemented. A temporary crown was then fitted to this tooth.

In view of the unstable position of the canine it was necessary to include a further abutment tooth in the bridge. The canine and first premolar were therefore prepared for full crown retainers.

Before an impression could be taken, certain precautions, usually necessary in cleft-palate patients, had to be observed. A piece of ribbon gauze was placed into the cleft and fistula, both palatally and labially and packed firmly into the defect.

After the impression had been taken, a temporary bridge was fitted to hold the abutment teeth in position. In cleft-palate patients temporary crowning of the abutment teeth and the fitting of a temporary denture to fill the space does not guarantee a stable position of the abutment teeth during construction of a bridge.

Finally, a four-unit bonded porcelain bridge was fitted.

Case 6.   Multiple resin-bonded bridges in oligodontia (Figure 10.6)
This young male patient had missing 3|23. Orthodontic treatment had already been carried out to approximate the other teeth present. No restorations were present and the patient was keen to avoid any tooth preparation. On both sides, the occlusion was such that a group function lateral occlusion could be developed without making the canine teeth unaesthetically short.

Minimal tooth preparation was undertaken and etched metal bridges were made. On the right side, the missing canine tooth was replaced with a cantilever design retained from the first premolar tooth.

On the left side the span was considered too long for a fixed–fixed design so two separate cantilever bridges were provided. At the request of the orthodontist, the second premolar tooth was included to prevent it from relapsing into its rotated position. The bridges were cemented under rubber dam.

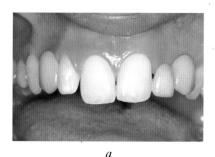

a

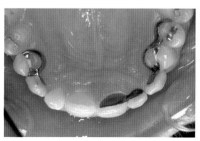

b

Figure 10.6 (a) Anterior view of completed bridges after 4 years of service. (b) Mirror view to demonstrate the design

The clinical pictures were taken at a four-year follow up. At that time it was decided to replace the anterior segment of the left side, not due to debonding but to improve the appearance with a longer pontic.

Case 7. Upper arch reconstruction (Figure 10.7)
The patient had undergone extensive restorative treatment over many years. A bridge was present replacing the upper left lateral incisor. The upper right second molar and upper left first molar had been missing for several years and the upper right first molar had recently been extracted. The upper right canine had been root filled. Several teeth showed marked mobility and radiographs indicated considerable bone loss. The occlusion was very heavy and there had been severe attrition with consequent loss of vertical height (Figure 10.7a). The loss of occlusal height was first treated by a removeable appliance, which was worn for several months to ensure that the correct vertical dimension had been established.

Bridge design. Since the patient's problems included both the replacement of missing teeth and the support of those remaining, a full arch bonded porcelain bridge was the treatment of choice. This extended from the upper left second molar to a cantilever pontic replacing the upper right first molar.

Preparations. At the first visit the upper right canine was prepared for a post and core, and full crown preparations were undertaken on the upper right premolars. Alignment was difficult and the pulp of the second premolar was exposed, so an immediate root filling was undertaken. A temporary bridge was inserted. At the second visit full crown preparations were undertaken on the upper left canine, premolars and second molar and a further temporary bridge fitted. At the third visit preparations were undertaken on the anterior teeth (Figure 10.7b), and a third temporary bridge fitted after full mouth impressions had been taken.

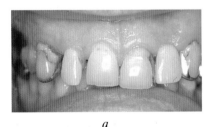

a

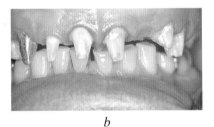

b

Figure 10.7 (a) Pre-operative view of the anterior teeth. (b) The prepared anterior teeth. (c) The temporary bridge. (d) Anterior view of the fitted bridge 5 years postoperatively. (Note the porcelain characterization used on the canines)

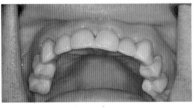

c

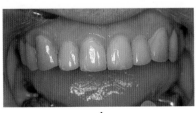

d

Temporary bridges. Acrylic temporary bridges were constructed from the model for the teeth prepared at each visit. A full arch temporary bridge was constructed on the model obtained from the impression (Figure 10.7c).

Try-in and cementation. The metal subframe was tried-in and, after minor adjustments, returned to the laboratory for the porcelain to be added. After cementation of the bridge (Figure 10.7d), the patient was asked to return on several occasions to ensure that the occlusion was fully adjusted, because large bridges can very easily cause minor alterations in the occlusion, which can be harmful and very uncomfortable to the patient.

Case 8.   Oral rehabilitation (Figure 10.8)
A male patient, aged 35, requested that his appearance be improved. He complained of absence of normal natural teeth, which had caused him considerable embarrassment over the past decade.

On examination, it was found that he had partial anodontia with retention of nine deciduous teeth, some of which were loose. The two upper central incisors and three lower permanent incisors were present. There were spaces between these anterior teeth and the posterior teeth, but these were too small for two pontics and too large for one pontic. This was discussed with the patient and it was suggested that orthodontic advice should be obtained. The patient agreed to fixed-appliance orthodontic treatment. This created spaces in the upper jaw for one pontic between the premolars on each side and two pontics each between the central incisors and first premolars. In the lower jaw adequate spaces were made for one incisor and both canines. In both jaws the molar teeth were not involved in the bridge work and both bridges extended from the second premolar on one side to the

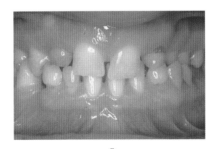

a

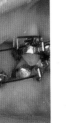

b

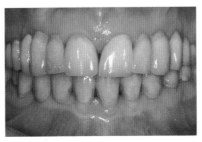

c

Figure 10.8 (a) A 35-year-old male with oligodontia and retained deciduous teeth. (b) Nine months later during the orthodontic treatment to create spaces for pontics of the correct size. (c) Three years after the start of treatment. Metal–ceramic bridges in both the upper and lower jaws

second premolar on the other side. In the upper jaw, four premolars and two central incisors were the abutment teeth to carry six pontics. In the lower jaw, four premolars and three incisors were the abutment teeth to carry three pontics.

After completion of the orthodontic treatment, intermediate acrylic bridges were prepared from study casts. The upper jaw was treated first and the premolars and incisors of one side were prepared for full, bonded porcelain crowns, followed by the preparation of the other side. After fitting the intermediate upper bridge the lower jaw was prepared. However, as the teeth had very small clinical crowns great care was necessary to avoid overpreparation. In view of this, preparation of the premolars on one side was followed by preparation of the premolars on the other side and finally the anterior teeth were prepared.

The three groups of teeth were prepared in separate sessions for full, bonded porcelain crowns and the lower intermediate bridge was fitted. After adjustments to the occlusion and other minor adjustments to improve the appearance of these two intermediate bridges, impressions were taken for a study cast to assist the technician in the construction of the permanent bridges.

After an interval of a few weeks to allow the patient to get used to the bridges, the intermediate bridges were removed and impressions were taken in polyether for the permanent bridges.

The instructions to the technician included a request for metal occlusal surfaces because of the lack of room for porcelain in this area, adequate interproximal spaces for cleaning, small contact areas for the pontics of the lower anterior regions and one-piece bridge work in both jaws to utilize a cross-arch splinting effect. This was considered important because of the amount of orthodontic movement of the abutment teeth in the recent past. Both bridges were fitted early one morning two weeks following the final impressions. They were not cemented. The patient was asked to have a meal and return later the same day for cementation. This short trial period allowed the bridges to settle down and this technique has a place in bridge work for selected patients. The whole treatment period including the orthodontics covered just over three years.

Case 9.   The use of an implant to replace a missing incisor tooth in a case with spacing (Figure 10.9)
The upper right central incisor tooth in this patient had to be lost due to resorption of the root. Unfortunately the adjacent teeth were unrestored and spacing was present on both sides of the tooth. A resin-bonded bridge in this situation would have been unsatisfactory. An implant fixture was therefore placed in the region of the tooth six weeks after its extraction.

Following osseo-integration after six months a crown was fitted to replace the missing tooth of the correct dimensions to maintain the natural spacing.

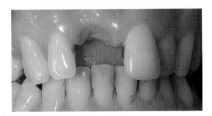

a

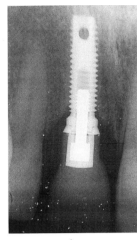

b

Figure 10.9 (a) Missing incisor
tooth. (Note the large potential
pontic space.) (b) Radiograph
showing fully integrated fixture.
(c) The fixture head *in situ*.
(d) The completed crown

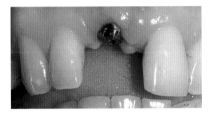

c

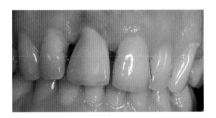

d

Chapter 11

Maintenance, failures and repair

Maintenance

The value of correct oral hygiene has already been well demonstrated in Chapter 2, and the importance of a high standard of maintenance by patient and dentist cannot be over emphasized. It is to be hoped that any crown or bridge placed will have a life expectancy of at least a decade and with a high level of maintenance, restorations are often seen surviving for 20 or 30 years.

Following cementation, the patient should be instructed in particular oral hygiene procedures necessary because of the restoration. For example, a crown needs brushing and flossing just as a sound tooth, but the position of the margins and the particular need for care in cleaning should be demonstrated to the patient. A mirror and good lighting are essential.

If a bridge has been placed, then particular care needs to be taken of the proximal area between the retainer and pontic. The patient will not be able to use dental floss in the conventional manner and the use of a floss threader or Superfloss should be demonstrated and then the patient encouraged to copy the technique in the surgery.

For any extensive restorations fitted, it is important that the patient be reviewed 1 to 2 weeks post-cementation so that the efficiency of cleaning can be assessed and any corrections made.

Patients who find difficulty with dental floss should have interproximal bottle brushes demonstrated as an alternative. Obviously if extensive bridge work has been fitted in a mouth that cannot be well-maintained, it is much more likely to fail and perhaps should not have been started. If there is a high decay rate or a decreased salivary flow, dietary advice should be given and the use of daily fluoride rinses (0.05%) are to be encouraged.

Athletes and patients with a tendency to brux should be provided with a suitable guard appliance.

The patient should be asked to return for review if any symptoms develop, mobility is felt or for some reason the restoration feels different from when cemented. This is often a sign that a problem is developing and action is best taken quickly.

Review appointments
These are made regularly dependant upon the amount and complexity of treatment, the caries rate and the standard or oral hygiene. This will normally be every 6 months.

The restoration is examined with a sharp probe to detect if marginal deficiencies or caries are present. Mobility of the tooth must be determined and/or mobility of the restoration relative to the tooth. This is a particular problem in bridges with multiple abutments. Pressure is applied to each retainer in turn looking for movement, and saliva movement or 'bubbling' from around the margins of the restoration. Gentle occlusal force should also be applied in the connector region. 'Bubbling' around retainers is an indication of trouble and must be investigated further.

A periodontal evaluation is carried out in the conventional manner and any loss of attachment noted. Bleeding on probing indicates active disease and the patient will need to be encouraged in better cleaning.

Periodic radiographic examination of crowns and bridges is essential. If there is any sign of marginal discrepancy, mobility or symptoms, a long-cone periapical radiograph of the abutment tooth is necessary. For routine checks, a bite-wing radiograph is adequate and these will be necessary every 2 to 3 years dependant upon the condition of the mouth. Patients at high risk from dental disease require radiographs more often.

If mobility is discovered, but there has been no decementation, the presence of periodontal pocketing should be determined and the occlusion checked, in case excessive loads are the cause.

Failures and repair

An objective evaluation of an existing restoration is necessary before coming to the conclusion that it is defective and requires either repair or replacement.

What constitutes a failure? Are failures absolute or are there degrees of failure? There are, of course, minor failures, which are a matter of opinion and could possibly be left without immediate repair or replacement, and there are obvious failures where repair or replacement is essential to avoid further damage to the dentition. Every crown or bridge failure presents a challenge. Each case is different and therefore of special interest to the clinician. Throughout this handbook, the emphasis is on simple inlays, crowns and bridges, and a discussion of complicated replacement of extensive multiple abutment bridges is not appropriate. Furthermore, it is impossible to say how long a tooth with a crown or bridge should last, failure may occur at any time. Loss of pulp vitality, for instance, may occur years after cementing a bridge and may be the end result of a chronic inflammation and a degenerating pulp beneath an otherwise intact bridge. If the cement seal is intact and if the retainer margins are caries-free, successful endodontic treatment may be carried out through the occlusal surface of the retainer without removing the bridge.

Reasons for failure

The principles of bridge design are mainly empirical and depend on the avoidance of factors known to cause failures. Therefore, it is important to isolate and analyse the causes of failure.

Figure 11.1 (a) A gold crown on a lower molar tooth. The crown is overextended distally and has an overhang resulting in food packing, which was aggravated by the lack of a contact point. (b) Some months later, a large carious lesion on the distal surface. (c) Root canal treatment completed and a new crown supported by a post

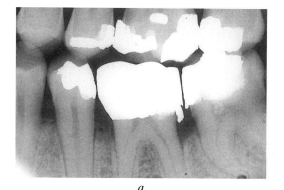

a

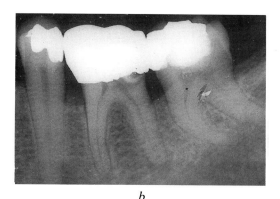

b

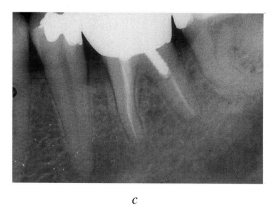

c

Caries. The most common reason for failure of crown or bridge work is caries (Figure 11.1). This can be due to poor oral hygiene, diet, poor dentistry or poor design or fit of the crown or bridge. Caries is a common problem with multiple retainer bridges when just one of several retainers becomes debonded.

Periodontal breakdown. Poorly-executed crown and bridge work with margins encroaching on the periodontal tissues causes stagnation and plaque accumulation and will result in gingival inflammation.

Periapical inflammation. This can result from poor or faulty preparation of abutment teeth, deep caries or large restorations.

Loss of a proximal contact. This may result if the occlusion is poorly restored, and can cause food packing in the approximal spaces, inflammation of the periodontal ligament and possibly further drifting of the abutment tooth. The end result of this can be pain, inflammation and a change in the occlusion with further complications.

Cementation. Cementation failures can be due to the wrong cement being used, faulty cementation techniques or loosening of the retainer because of inadequate retention. Inadequate retention can be due to incorrect abutment preparation or faulty bridge design.

Mechanical breakdown of components. Fracture of an all-metal bridge usually occurs at the joint but even this is relatively uncommon. A metal–ceramic bridge can also fracture at this place because of an inadequate thickness of the metal joint, although most small metal–ceramic bridges are cast as one unit. Fracture of a porcelain facing is not uncommon and is usually due to trauma such as contact sport accidents or biting on a hard object. Overbuilt porcelain unsupported by the metal substructure in a metal–ceramic crown may fracture because of a cohesive failure within the porcelain (Figure 11.2).

Flexion of gold retainers. This is uncommon with the use of harder gold alloys. It can happen when a retainer is too thin or covers only part of the tooth. Occlusal stresses may then produce flexion of the retainer with subsequent breakdown of the cement seal.

Occlusion. A faulty occlusion caused by either the new crown or bridge or by a change in the occlusion due to other restorations, can also be the cause of failure.

Wear and tear. Not to be forgotten is the fact that a crown or bridge can fail because of wear and tear over a period of time and this is usually nobody's fault.

Single unit failures

All-porcelain crowns. In spite of periodic advertisements for 'newer and better' restorative materials for this purpose, it is impossible to guarantee a

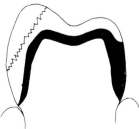

Figure 11.2 Overbuilt porcelain unsupported by gold may allow cohesive failure within the porcelain facing

repair of porcelain crowns except as a short-term temporary measure. Severely fractured or chipped all-porcelain crowns must therefore be replaced by a new crown. This also gives the operator an opportunity to consider the possible need for a different or more suitable type of crown or to modify the preparation.

Gold crowns. These do not fracture very often but general wear and tear can cause a perforation occlusally, leaving the core of the abutment tooth exposed. In this situation, if the perforation is small, the hole in the metal is enlarged and the new edges carefully explored to ensure that caries has not undermined the perforation. Any caries present is removed and the cavity filled with a suitable material. The most commonly used material for this purpose is amalgam, although composites and glass–ionomer cements are good alternatives. Marginal caries must be removed and if access is difficult, part of the crown or bridge retainer can be cut out to facilitate the removal of caries. Gingival surgery is sometimes needed to obtain access to marginal caries.

Metal–ceramic crowns. The most common defect is the loss of part of the porcelain veneer. In the posterior region of the mouth, if appearance is not important and the exposed metal surface is not unacceptable clinically or aesthetically, this can often be left without replacement or repair after smoothing down the rough edges.

In the anterior region of the mouth replacement of lost porcelain is sometimes possible using a resin-bonding agent and a light-cured composite material. This type of repair is limited to small areas not exposed to heavy occlusal forces.

When a large part of the labial surface is lost it is sometimes possible to remove all the porcelain from the metal substructure as well as some of the metal from the labial and palatal surfaces. An impression of the remaining parts of the crown is taken and followed by the construction of a 'sleeve crown'. This type of repair/replacement is usually reserved for a damaged bridge unit and will be described in detail in the next section.

Bridge failures

As bridges are several single units soldered or cast into one unit the defects and reasons for failure of any of the single units described above apply also to bridge units.

However, because of the greater area of periodontal tissue involved, as well as the greater area of occlusion and the potentially damaging effect of leverage, there are additional problems and possibilities of failure.

Loss of retention. This is a common cause of failure because of leverage and unequal occlusal loads on different parts of the bridge. A loose retainer causes rapid destruction of the abutment core, which is usually made up of dentine without its protective enamel cover. It is the saliva, plaque and pumping action of the loose retainer that are responsible for caries leading to very rapid destruction of the abutment tooth. For this reason, a loose

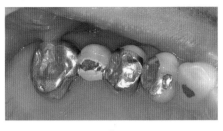

a

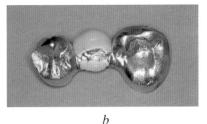

b

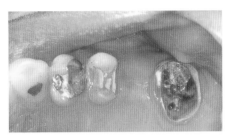

c

Figure 11.3 (a) A three-unit fixed bridge that failed.
(b) A perforation on the occluso-palatal aspect of the full gold molar retainer is clearly visible.
(c) Almost the entire clinical crown of the molar abutment tooth has been destroyed by caries

retainer of a bridge must not be left for treatment at some later date but treated immediately. It is better for the tooth to have no cover than a loose cover (Figure 11.3).

Loss of retention is often due to poor clinical dentistry. When abutment preparations lack near parallelism of opposing walls, or depend on cores that are too short and are subjected to adverse stresses during occlusion, the bridge is doomed to failure. The result is usually a break in the cement seal, caries and eventual damage to the pulp of the abutment tooth, as well as damage to other abutment teeth of the bridge.

Caries. When construction of a bridge is recommended, the dentist usually takes into account the patient's suitability and has given all the necessary advice regarding plaque control and general maintenance of a bridge. However, from time to time, bridges are made for patients who are not totally suitable and furthermore, they do sometimes change their habits and attitudes. Plaque control and diet may therefore change. Evidence of at least a reasonable oral hygiene is therefore necessary.

Design faults. There are design faults that may cause the destruction of the supporting tissues of a bridge (Figure 11.4). For instance, inadequate spacing between the retainer or pontic units of a bridge, and inadequate room for interdental papillae, will cause stagnation areas, food traps and

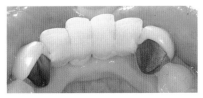

a

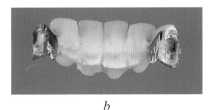

b

Figure 11.4 (a) A six-unit lower anterior metal–ceramic bridge with little regard for access for cleaning devices and the maintenance of oral hygiene.
(b) The bridge has been removed by sectioning the retainers. (Note the faulty pontic design, which was the cause of the problem)

soft tissue damage, as well as caries. Overextended crowns will lead to similar problems. The remedy is obvious. Overextended crowns or retainers must not be accepted, no matter how much pressure is on the dentist to complete treatment in the time estimated or promised.

The 'sleeve crown'

When a considerable portion of the porcelain facing is lost from the labial or incisal surface of a retainer or pontic it is often possible to effect a repair by a replacement of much of that unit without removal of the bridge.

The porcelain facing is removed with a diamond bur and some of the metal substructure from the labial surface. Porcelain as well as metal are removed from the incisal third of the palatal surface. This is a simple procedure when the damaged unit is a pontic but when the unit is a retainer and the underlying pulp has to be considered, caution is necessary to avoid damage to the abutment tooth. A common mistake is the removal of too little porcelain and metal.

An impression is taken of this and the two adjacent units. The technician is then asked to make a metal–ceramic crown that will have two surfaces instead of the usual four. This sleeve crown is then cemented in the usual way. If too little porcelain is removed from the original unit, the new sleeve crown will feel slightly bulky. The appearance, however, should be as good as the original bridge unit (Figure 11.5).

As previously mentioned, small porcelain fractures can be repaired as a temporary measure (Figure 11.6).

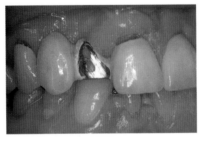

a

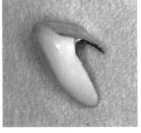

b

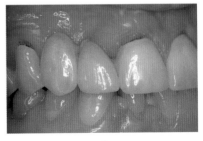

c

Figure 11.5 (a) A three-unit metal–ceramic bridge that had the damaged labial porcelain of the pontic removed and prepared for a sleeve crown. (b) The sleeve crown before cementation. (c) The repaired bridge

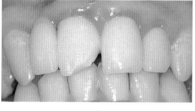

a

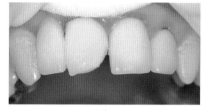

b

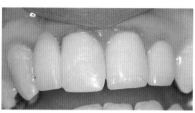

c

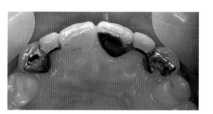

d

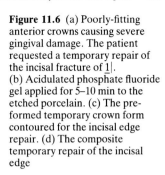

Figure 11.6 (a) Poorly-fitting anterior crowns causing severe gingival damage. The patient requested a temporary repair of the incisal fracture of 1|. (b) Acidulated phosphate fluoride gel applied for 5–10 min to the etched porcelain. (c) The preformed temporary crown form contoured for the incisal edge repair. (d) The composite temporary repair of the incisal edge

Figure 11.7 Debonding of the retainer of an upper central incisor has resulted in decalcification and caries in the cingulum area. (Note the failed wing has been removed)

Resin-bonded bridges

Retainer debonding is the commonest cause of failure of resin-bonded bridge work (Figure 11.7). This may be caused by inappropriate case selection, inadequate tooth preparation, errors in bonding or occlusal interferences. The failure may occur at the metal–resin interface, enamel–resin interface or cohesive failure in the resin cement. The cause of failure should be identified as this will determine the treatment required. If the fault can be corrected (e.g. elimination of occlusal interference) then the bridge may be re-cemented. Otherwise it will have to be remade to correct any faults in design.

Greying of anterior abutment incisal edges may result when there is excessive extension of the metal framework on thin incisor teeth (Figure 11.8). Therefore thin anterior crowns may change in colour following cementation of a resin-bonded retainer because the translucency is lost. As

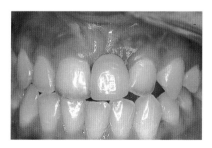

Figure 11.8 A resin-bonded bridge fitted to replace the upper central incisor caused the grey appearance of the tips of the abutment teeth

the shade of the pontic will have been chosen before cementation, the final appearance will be that of variously shaded teeth and, in spite of its technical excellence, the bridge will be deemed a failure because of the unsatisfactory appearance. Gold coating of the metal framework and opaque luting cements are only a partial solution to this problem.

Removing crowns and bridges

Before the removal of a crown is attempted the possible need for a temporary crown must be remembered and provision for this should be made (see Chapter 4). Furthermore, it is important to remember that bridges, crowns and, particularly, inlays are small objects and that during their removal the patient's airway must be protected at all times. Sometimes it is helpful to alter the position of the chair and have the patient sitting upright.

The removal of crowns
Gold crowns can be removed relatively easily. Various instruments can be used but the Morell crown/bridge remover is probably one of the most suitable (Figure 11.9). If this fails to loosen the crown a small hole is made in the occlusal surface and a pair of pliers, similar to orthodontic molar band removers, are used. When pressure is applied the crown usually loosens. If all else fails, a small cut is made along the buccal surface of the crown and a chisel is applied to the surface cuts. Gentle lever action usually breaks the cement seal. The seal can also sometimes be broken by the application of an ultrasonic scaler to the crown margins.

Figure 11.9 The Morell crown remover. The sliding weight can be replaced by a heavier one, and the attachment for application to the cervical margin of the retainer is also replaceable

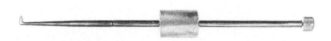

A similar method can sometimes be used for metal–ceramic crowns but the porcelain veneer usually fractures and the patient should be warned of this before crown removal is attempted. It is unusual for a metal–ceramic crown to be removed without fracture of the porcelain.

Porcelain jacket crowns, as mentioned above, cannot usually be removed without damage and most operators do not even try to remove one intact. A long, tapered diamond instrument may be used to cut through the incisal and labial faces of the crown. This will split it and the pieces are removed by leverage with a small, flat plastic instrument.

The removal of posts
The success of post removal depends much on its length beyond the core. Several instruments are available for the removal of posts that cannot be easily removed with an ordinary pair of pliers. The Masseran kit was designed for the removal of fractured posts well-embedded in the canal. It works on the principle of enlarging the canal around the post and thereby loosening it (Figure 11.10).

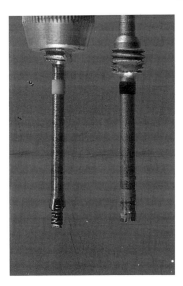

Figure 11.10 Two hollow tube drill bits from the Masseran kit. The left bit has a fractured post still in the tube immediately after removal from the root canal

The removal of bridges

As is the case with crowns, bridge removal must be explained to the patient in great detail. It is important to make clear that bridge removal might result in failure or complications necessitating extraction of a tooth, or involvement of additional teeth and a new bridge. Unless this is understood and accepted by the patient, bridge removal should not be attempted.

If the bridge is to be destroyed or the abutment tooth extracted, the removal is not difficult. Sectioning the various units either through the pontic or the joints will facilitate the removal. Sectioning the bridge by making cuts along a vertical surface of a retainer has its difficulties. Care must be taken not to damage the abutment tooth by cutting into its core. A diamond instrument is used to cut through the porcelain facing. The metal is then prised away from the tooth to break the cement seal.

Great care is necessary when a bridge is to be removed intact so that it can be modified and replaced. The Morell bridge remover has a tip that is hooked onto the crown margin and operates by the movement of a sliding weight along a handle producing a tapping action when the weight reaches a metal stop. This is often used with great success. When it has broken the cement seal of one retainer it is moved along to the next unit for the same action. Alternatively, bridges can sometimes be removed by threading dental floss or thin copper wire through the proximal spaces and looping it around a strong metal rod held horizontally at 90° to the long axis of the abutment teeth about 15 cm from the bridge. Two or three wires are sufficient. A sharp tap on the metal rod will loosen the bridge. This method is dramatic and not without risk. The patient must be warned beforehand what to expect.

Resin-bonded bridges are much simpler to remove. A tap on a chisel placed at the metal and tooth junction should loosen the bridge. Sometimes it is necessary to section it before using a chisel. Ultrasonic scalers have also been used with some success for the removal of these bridges.

In view of the complications that may arise when a bridge has failed, it is

Figure 11.11 A lateral perforation caused by a post. This type of damage can sometimes be salvaged without removal of the bridge by surgical repair. The patient was surprised to hear that the bridge was not in perfect order.

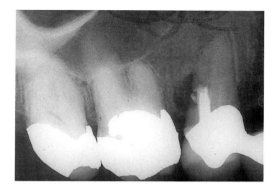

wise to consider the possible need for the removal of the bridge during the design stage. A large bridge should, whenever possible, be so designed that one section can be removed, if necessary, without disturbance of the other sections. The replacement of a part of a bridge is often possible by careful sectioning of the units in the pontic areas. The new replacement section is then fitted to the remaining sections, which are modified to act as substructures.

Failures of crowns and bridges are not always obvious and the need for repair must be shown and explained to the patient (Figure 11.11). The problem arises when the patient believes the bridge or crown to be good and functional. It is usually wise before removing the evidence, in other words, the failed bridge or crown, to take radiographs, study casts and if possible, photographs.

Suggestions for further reading

Albers H. F. (1990) *Impressions — a text for selection of materials and techniques.* Santa Rosa, Alto Books

Banks R. G. (1990) Conservative posterior ceramic restorations: a literature review. *J Prosthet Dent* **63**, 619–26

Baylis M. A. and Williams J. D. (1986) Using the twin-stage Occluder with a functionally generated pathway record. *Quintess Dental Technol* **10**, 361–5

Capp J. N. (1985) The diagnostic use of provisional restorations. *Restorative Dent* **1**, 92–8

Fagin M. D. (1981) Restoration of endodontically treated teeth. *Int J Perio Restor Dent* **1**(3), 8–29

Ibbetson R. J. and Setchell D. J. (1989) Treatment of the worn dentition. *Dental Update* Vol. **16**, **6**, 247–53 and 300–7

Jordan R. E. (1986) *Esthetic Composite Bonding — Techniques and Materials.* Burlington, B. C. Decker

Kantorowicz G. F. (1971) The repair and removal of bridges. *Dent Practitioner* **21**, 341–6

Kantorowicz G. F. (1975) Bridge prostheses for cleft palate patients: an analysis. *Br Dent J* **139**, 91–7

Kayser A. F. (1989) The shortened dental arch: a therapeutic concept in reduced dentitions and certain high risk groups. *Int J Perio Restor Dent* **9**, 427–49

Kidd E. A. M. and Smith B. G. N. (1990) *Pickard's Manual of Operative Dentistry.* 6th edn, Oxford, Oxford Medical

McLean J. W. (1979) *The Science and Art of Dental Ceramics.* Vol. 1, Chicago, Quintessence

McLean J. W. (1980) *The Science and Art of Dental Ceramics.* Vol. 2, Chicago, Quintessence

Nicholls E. (1984) *Endodontics.* 3rd edn, Bristol, J. Wright & Sons

Nyman S. and Ericsson I. (1982) The capacity of reduced periodontal tissues to support fixed bridgework. *J Clin Periodont* **9**, 409–14

Pameijer J. H. N. (1985) *Periodontal and occlusal factors in crown and bridge procedures.* Dental Center for Postgraduate Courses, Amsterdam

Prieskel H. W. (1979) *Precision Attachments in Dentistry.* 3rd edn, London, Kimpton

Reuter J. E. and Brose M. O. (1984) Failures in full crown retained dental bridges. *Br Dent J* **157**, 61–3

Roberts D. H. (1970) The failure of retainers in bridge prostheses. *Br Dent J* **128**, 117–24

Shillingburg H. T., Jacobi R. and Brackett S. E. (1987) *Fundamentals of tooth preparations — for cast metal and porcelain restorations.* Chicago, Quintessence

Smith B. G. N. (1990) *Planning and Making Crowns and Bridges.* 2nd edn, Martin Dunitz

Tay W. M. (1992) *Resin-bonded Bridges: A Practitioner's Guide.* Martin Dunitz

Warren K. and Capp N. (1990) A review of principles and techniques for making interocclusal records for mounting working casts. *Int J Prosth* **3(4)**, 341–8

Wilson H. J., McLean J. W. and Brown D. (1988) Dental materials and their clinical applications. *Br Dent J*

Wohlwend A., Strub J. R. and Scharer P. (1989) Metal ceramic and all porcelain restorations: current considerations. *Int J Prosthodont* **2**, 13–26

Zarb G. A. *et al.* (1978) *Prosthodontic treatment for partially edentulous patients.* St. Louis, C. V. Mosby

Index